Fractal: About Community Acupuncture

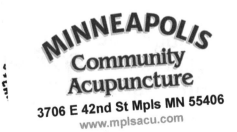

MINNEAPOLIS
Community
Acupuncture
3706 E 42nd St Mpls MN 55406
www.mplsacu.com

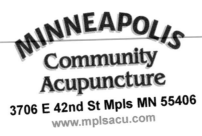

MINNEAPOLIS
Community
Acupuncture
3706 E 42nd St Mpls MN 55406
www.mplsacu.com

Fractal:

About Community Acupuncture

By Lisa Rohleder, L.Ac.

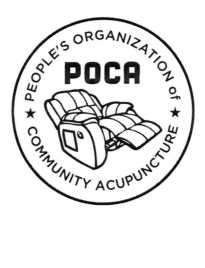

In memory of Chico Senn

Thank you to all the members of the POCA Cooperative who made this book possible, especially Gloria Jacobs, Wade Phillips, Sean Nolan, and Annie Tessar.

"What do we live for, if it is not to make life less difficult for each other?"
–George Eliot

Table of Contents

Prologue: The Spoiler

How do you know if you want to read this book? You might never have heard of community acupuncture, and you're wondering if it's worth your time to find out more about it. You should be able to figure that out by reading this prologue, which sums up the story by starting at the end. Community acupuncture is a Thing now, a significant Thing to a lot of people, because it helps them. But it wasn't always a Thing. This is the story of how community acupuncture got to the point of being a Thing that needed to have books written about it (and documentaries made, and newspaper articles published, but that all comes later).

Acupuncture is a Thing that works. Nobody really knows why; it is very, very old. Mainstream culture in the US doesn't quite know what to do with acupuncture. Nonetheless, it is a Thing that works. It works for a very long list of problems: allergies, asthma, anxiety, all kinds of pain, depression, poor digestion, chronic health conditions, and stress. It doesn't always fix these problems entirely, but more often than not, it helps. Sometimes it helps spectacularly – so much so, that it is usually worth trying.

Unfortunately, a lot of people can't try it, because it's become too expensive.

Once upon a time – for much of its history – acupuncture was a very cheap therapy, used by poor people. It was practiced in a group setting, so if you got acupuncture, you probably got it in a room with other people who were getting acupuncture at the same time. This changed when acupuncture began to be practiced widely in the West. It became an expensive therapy, marketed to people with a lot of disposable income. Also, acupuncture practice became individual: if you got acupuncture, you probably got it alone in a little cubicle.

At the same time, it became very hard for acupuncturists to make a living. If you tried very hard to treat mostly rich people, you might be successful. By far the best way to practice acupuncture, though, was to have another source of income (like a spouse with a good job) so that you didn't have to worry about making money.

I went to acupuncture school when I was very young and I didn't know what I was getting into. The family I come from is not rich; they're a mix of working-class/working poor/just barely lower middle-class. I fell in love with another acupuncturist. Neither of us wanted to get a good, non-acupuncture job; both of us wanted to be acupuncturists. I also wanted to be able to treat people like my family. I was in big trouble.

The solution I came up with was to redesign the business model and to go back to what acupuncture looked like when it was a therapy for poor people. My partner and I opened a clinic in a working-class neighborhood where we treated people all together in a big room instead of individually in little cubicles, and we called it "Community Acupuncture." It worked. We made a living. Our neighbors got a lot of acupuncture.

That was over a decade ago. Now community acupuncture is a Thing. There are hundreds of clinics that do acupuncture this way and hundreds of thousands of people getting acupuncture who previously couldn't afford it. Community acupuncture seems like a good Thing, a Thing that should grow and be available to millions of people because, after all, it is a Thing that works. Health care is an expensive, dysfunctional mess. Community acupuncture is cheap, simple, and effective.

Those of us who care about community acupuncture have been trying to make it available to as many people as possible. This is hard because acupuncture is not a Thing our culture understands. This is not just because acupuncture comes from Asia and involves theories about Yin and Yang. It's because acupuncture is quiet and uncomplicated and not designed to make a profit.

This book tells the story of how community acupuncture became a Thing, and what kind of Thing it is, but most importantly, explains how we think more people could get it. Because that is the most important thing.

Community acupuncture, as a Thing and as a story, is like a repeating pattern. Another word for a repeating pattern is *fractal*. The same elements keep showing up. We want you to be able to see the whole pattern – and even if you are not all that interested in acupuncture, the pattern suggests some notable things about business, human nature, and our society in general.

When we first opened our clinic, lots of people told us, "This won't work." Patients won't want to get acupuncture in a group, because they want to have their acupuncturist and their healing space all to themselves. They don't care if somebody else can afford to get acupuncture; they only care about themselves. This will never be a real Thing, it will only be one tiny little clinic that is run in a funny way.

It turned out that some patients think like this, but a whole lot don't. Many patients don't mind sharing their acupuncturist and their healing space. Many patients do genuinely care about whether or not other people can afford to get acupuncture.

When we first tried to get other acupuncturists to think about using our model, lots of people told us, "This won't work." Acupuncturists don't care if people can afford to get acupuncture; they only care about how much money they can make. They want to have acupuncture all to themselves. Community acupuncture will never be a Thing.

It turned out that some acupuncturists are like this, but a whole lot aren't. Many acupuncturists do care about whether people can afford to get acupuncture. Many acupuncturists find tremendous joy in helping as many people as possible.

When we created the Community Acupuncture Network, an organization for community acupuncturists, lots of people told us, "This won't work." Community acupuncture may be a Thing for a few acupuncturists, but it will never be more than a handful. Acupuncturists are competitive and secretive. They won't help each other; they won't share information; they don't care if other acupuncturists can make a living. They want to keep what they know all to themselves. Acupuncture organizations fail because acupuncturists can't work together.

It turned out that some acupuncture organizations are like this, but the Community Acupuncture Network was not. Many acupuncturists did help each other. They did share information. And, with each other's support, a hundred or so community acupuncture clinics got off the ground.

When we realized that we needed to include patients in a more formal way, we created a cooperative called the **People's Organization of Community Acupuncture.**[1] A lot of people told us, "This won't work." Nobody's going to join a

---

[1] http://www.pocacoop.com

cooperative. They don't care about the future of acupuncture; they don't want to think about how the economics of acupuncture can be sustainable. They're not going to give their time, their attention, and their energy to a co-op; they want to keep their time, attention and energy all to themselves. All that people care about is whether it is a Thing that is available to them when they feel like using it. They don't care if anybody else can have it in the future.

You see the pattern.

We did a lot of work to make community acupuncture into a Thing. It was fun work, because it was creative and hopeful. Health care in this country has been constructed to appeal to the worst impulses in people: fear, greed, and the desire to evade responsibility for ourselves and each other. Everybody knows it's broken. It's discouraging to try to fix it. But community acupuncture is the opposite of fear and greed; community acupuncture is all about the willingness to take responsibility for ourselves and each other. At every step of the way, working on it has made us feel whole, more connected to ourselves and to each other.

Community acupuncture is a Thing now because a lot of people were able to see past *what's in it for me?* A lot of people wanted to share instead of keeping it all to themselves. At each stage of the pattern, we had to push past resistance. *Why are you dropping your prices? You'll never get anywhere that way. Why don't you just focus on your own clinic? You can't make any money off other community acupuncture clinics, so why put energy into helping them? You'll never get anywhere that way. Why put all this energy into trying to make a cooperative, into trying to make infrastructure for community acupuncture? You'll never get anywhere that way.* Our culture has a very hard time thinking about things collectively instead of individually.

Community acupuncture is a Thing because a lot of us are stubborn and refused to listen. We decided that it made more sense to think about acupuncture collectively, not just individually. And it turned out that we did get somewhere: we got to a much better place collectively AND individually. We got to the point that hundreds of thousands of people could get as much acupuncture as they wanted. We got to the point that a lot of acupuncturists could make a living. We made clinics and we made jobs. We're going to make an acupuncture school.

This is where you come in.

If community acupuncture is a good thing for you, if it is a benefit to you as an individual, whether you're a patient or an acupuncturist, that's because a whole lot of other people didn't just think about what's in it for them. So now we are asking you to think about more than just *what's in it for me?* Yes, you can use community acupuncture however you want; you don't have to care about it as a Thing if you don't want to. But please remember that the only reason it's here for you is that is a lot of other people DID care.

So what can you do? Take the time to read this book so that you can see the whole pattern. When you get acupuncture, think about all the other people who need it. Get connected to the rest of us and join the **People's Organization of Community Acupuncture**. You can help us make this Thing more of a Thing, for a lot more people.

Introduction

In 2006, I wrote and self-published a book titled *The Remedy, Integrating Acupuncture into American Health Care*. I had an idea that I was really passionate about and I thought I'd toss it out into the world to see what would happen. In the past seven years, I've learned a lot about what happens when an idea that had mostly only lived in my head (and a few other people's heads) starts to take shape out in the world where everyone can see it.

It's fascinating watching an idea become reality. It takes on substance a little at a time; it fills out and gathers dimension. It solidifies and accumulates detail, edges, aspects. It sprouts tendrils in unexpected places. In the case of this particular idea, it turned out that when it became reality, it took the shape of a fractal.

What's a fractal? If you've ever eaten broccoli or cauliflower you've encountered a fractal (and ingested it, to boot).

A fractal is a complex, repeating pattern, in which every part is a miniature copy of the whole. Fractals are everywhere in nature: broccoli is one of the most familiar. (Romanesco broccoli is one of the most spectacular.) When you cut up a head of broccoli, you can see that the individual florets are the same shape as the stalk; it's the same pattern repeated at different scales. Snowflakes work the same way, as do leaves, blood vessels, lightning, ferns, peacock feathers, rivers, and mountain ranges. The initial pattern appears to be random but becomes remarkably consistent as it repeats itself at different scales.

What does affordable acupuncture have to do with rivers, mountain ranges, ferns and broccoli? And why should you care? This book is going to try to answer those questions.

In *The Remedy* I first wrote about community acupuncture. Since then it has turned out to be a kind of living organism and a fractal, though I would never have realized it if Cris Monteiro, my friend and fellow community acupuncturist, hadn't pointed it out.

In 2006 there were a handful of community acupuncturists, treating about a thousand patients. Now there are hundreds of community acupuncturists, treating hundreds of thousands of patients. If you read the original *Remedy*, you can see the basic pattern, or a sketchy outline of it, but there's no indication of how the pattern would repeat itself over and over until it became a flourishing three-dimensional fractal — or what that might mean for acupuncturists, patients and health care.

One of the ironies of the original *Remedy* was that I wrote about community acupuncture from an individual perspective. The community acupuncture model came into being in part because I had some very specific needs, based on my history and my circumstances, and that was what most of the original *Remedy* was about. It turned out that the model met other people's needs even when their history and circumstances were different; it opened up access to acupuncture for all kinds of different people. In the years that followed, we discovered that community acupuncture doesn't work very well when you approach it from a narrowly individual vantage point. If you focus on one broccoli floret in isolation, you can't see the fractal. It came into being because of the needs of an individual, but its growth wasn't about any one individual at all.

So we're putting the original *Remedy* out of print, and this is the replacement. This book is for anyone who is interested in the community acupuncture movement – patients, potential patients, acupuncturists, people who design organizations, or curious onlookers. This book does not have a lot of technical information about acupuncture; if you are an acupuncturist looking for that and how it relates to community acupuncture, there are two books that might help: *Acupuncture Is Like Noodles* (2009) and *Tungsten, or Acupuncture in Large Quantities* (2013 pending). More good information can be found in the online forums of the **POCA Cooperative**.

This book is about the community acupuncture movement itself and its fractal growth. After seven years, the original *Remedy* was desperately outdated, in part because it was just a proposal for something that is now actually happening. This book updates the original *Remedy* and incorporates elements of other things I've written over the last seven years (blog posts, conference speeches, and articles) to give a better sense of the big picture.

As community acupuncturists say at the end of a treatment when we're taking the needles out and our patients are getting ready to go back out into the world: I hope it helps.

Why Acupuncture?

What is acupuncture? To answer that question as simply as possible, acupuncture is the millennia-old practice of inserting fine needles at specific points on the body for the purpose of cultivating health or alleviating symptoms.

Acupuncture is one of the oldest, simplest, and safest forms of health care in the world. Though no one knows exactly how it works, it seems to stimulate the body's self-healing and self-regulating mechanisms. This means that it can treat a wide range of problems, without causing major negative side effects. In fact, the main side effects of acupuncture are all positive; no matter why someone is seeking treatment or where an acupuncturist places the needles, acupuncture seems to produce similar overall benefits: increased energy, reduced stress, lower levels of inflammation, better sleep, improved moods, and often, a general sense of well-being and relaxation.

This makes acupuncture particularly helpful to Americans in the 21st century, because we are some of the most stressed-out people in history.

Acupuncture is good for treating chronic problems, such as diabetes, hypertension and arthritis, which can be managed but very rarely reversed or cured. Some people speculate that acupuncture works by interfacing between the body's nervous system and the circulatory system, and certainly it seems to improve blood circulation in general. As a result, it can sometimes help patients with chronic disorders have a better quality of life and reduce their need for multiple medications. This is especially true for patients suffering from chronic pain, a condition which conventional medicine often struggles with. According to the Centers for Disease Control, the leading causes of death and disability in the US are chronic diseases. Recent studies suggest that chronic pain affects 25% or more of the population. There are a lot of people who could potentially benefit from acupuncture.

Just as acupuncture is good for ameliorating the effects of chronic disease, it is similarly effective at treating garden-variety problems such as headaches, back pain, joint stiffness, muscle tension and stress. Acupuncture theory suggests that many common physical and emotional problems result, simply, from "stagnation" – from things not moving well and not working together smoothly within a person. As a result, acupuncture is able to treat common problems without over-medicalizing them. Unlike conventional medicine, which relies heavily on diagnosis via expensive and invasive testing, and often leads to a prescription for pharmaceuticals, acupuncture can be a very simple solution to garden-variety problems. Just as acupuncture produces positive global effects on sleep, mood and energy, no matter where the acupuncturist puts the needles, acupuncture is good at getting things moving and getting things working together in situations where pain and tension are a result of stagnation and disharmony. Acupuncture might be able to resolve a case of poor digestion, or a strained low back, with nothing more than a series of simple treatments. Treatments typically look something like this: a person with a garden-variety problem shows up for acupuncture, explains the issue in a few sentences. The acupuncturist inserts some needles, and the person sits quietly for an hour or so while things get moving, and leaves feeling better. Repeat as needed. No MRIs required. Of course, if acupuncture doesn't help, it's appropriate to access the bigger guns of conventional medicine. But it's often a good thing for the individual, and for society as a whole, to be able to try a low-tech, non-invasive, inexpensive option first – especially when the principal side effect of that low-tech option is stress reduction.

Acupuncture is a good thing for 21st century Americans because it is very simple, both in its essence and its tools. What you need to provide acupuncture are sterile, hair-thin, disposable needles; a bio-hazard container, some cotton balls; and a quiet place for the person receiving acupuncture to rest. That's all: needles, cotton balls, and stillness. If your goals for the acupuncture you are providing are appropriately modest – to improve the quality of life for people suffering from chronic diseases or chronic pain, to resolve garden-variety problems like headaches and back pain, and to reduce the stress of living in 21st century America – you don't really need a conventional medical diagnosis. You just need to know where to put the needles and how to do it safely.

Simplicity and modesty notwithstanding, acupuncture can have amazing, transformative effects, not only for individuals but for families and even communities. Pain and stress, in all their various manifestations, may not be particularly complex, but nonetheless they have a great capacity to make people miserable. When one person in a family is struggling to manage his chronic pain, feeling irritable and exhausted and hopeless, everyone else is affected. When that one person starts feeling even a little better, having energy to help his kids with their homework or to be a supportive listener to his spouse or ultimately return to work, that positive change ripples outward to affect more and more people. Sometimes the effects of acupuncture are particularly potent and empowering because they don't involve drugs or surgery or much outside intervention at all; they can be an affirmation to people that their own internal resources are enough to make a difference in their lives. That can be very encouraging, all by itself.

Because acupuncture can improve people's quality of life in various low-key but substantial ways, the correct answer to the question of "How much acupuncture does someone need in order to treat ____ (insert name of problem)?" is "As much acupuncture as they want!" From a clinical perspective, that is what works best. If someone is suffering from a serious, chronic condition, including chronic pain, of course, you're looking at a whole lot of acupuncture. However, this is another way that acupuncture is simple: just as it uses people's internal resources to address their problems, the best way to determine how much acupuncture people need is to allow them to experiment with getting acupuncture, notice its impact on their quality of life, and let them make the decision themselves. There is no complex formula. People are different, and like other therapies, acupuncture helps them to different degrees. Similarly, acupuncture doesn't "interact" with other interventions. You can get acupuncture in conjunction with any other therapy.

Acupuncture's simplicity has made it difficult to deliver to the people who could benefit from it the most. It does not fit well into the health care system we have, which is designed around complex, expensive interventions that require elaborate diagnostic procedures. No insurance company on earth will pay for unlimited amounts of acupuncture for a patient with chronic pain – yet that's exactly what usually works best in the real world. Since needles, cotton balls and stillness are all you need – and needles are the most expensive part of the package, at about 2 cents per needle – what should acupuncture cost?

Acupuncture isn't like other kinds of health care, because its tools and its essence are so simple, and because it relies so much on the internal resources of the person receiving it. The structures and formulas that have been set up to support the delivery of other kinds of health care largely limit acupuncture or actively interfere with it. Acupuncture's effects are so global, so modest, and so wide-ranging that it's almost beneath scientific notice; it's hard for conventional medicine, with its focus on diagnosis, to be interested in something that works best for everything in general and nothing in particular. For people suffering from some manifestation of pain or stress, however, especially if it's interfering with their ability to live their lives, acupuncture's potential is fascinating. Relief without side effects, and without drugs? Many people have an acute, personal interest in that.

Acupuncture In The West

The origins of acupuncture are long lost and probably precede written records. One of the first books written about acupuncture was *The Yellow Emperor's Classic of Internal Medicine*, circa 200 BCE in China. In 1991, a well-preserved mummy with tattoos at, or near, a number of recognizable acupuncture points was discovered near the Austrian-Italian border. Archaeologists determined that the mummy, christened "The Iceman," died around 3300 BCE. Does this mean that acupuncture – or something like it – was practiced in Europe in the Bronze Age? As with so many other aspects of acupuncture, we don't know.

One thing we do know is that acupuncture, then and now, is well-traveled.[2] It is common throughout Asia, including China, Japan, Vietnam, and Korea. It has been practiced in Europe (not counting The Iceman) since the 1800s, and is practiced today in Latin America, Australia, and North America. Acupuncture first arrived in the United States in the 1800s by two different routes: through medical doctors who decided to try it after reading journal articles about French physicians who experimented with it, and through Chinese immigrants who practiced it in their own communities.[1] Acupuncture received widespread mainstream attention after Nixon's 1972 visit to China. James Reston, a *New York Times* reporter, needed an emergency appendectomy and received acupuncture for post-operative pain. He was so impressed with the results that he wrote an article about his experience[3]. In Asia, acupuncture has always been practiced in groups. Famous acupuncturists were revered for their ability to treat a

---

[2] *Needles, Herbs, Gods and Ghosts: China, Healing and the West to 1848*, Linda L. Barnes.

[3] http://www.acupuncture.com/testimonials/restonexp.htm

hundred patients a day, often in humble village settings. (Famous acupuncturists were not necessarily wealthy acupuncturists.) As China modernized, acupuncturists moved into busy, communal hospitals wards. Historically, an acupuncture treatment was a relatively cheap commodity.

The first American acupuncture schools and professional organizations were founded in the 1970s, and some states passed laws that legalized acupuncture and licensed practitioners. In the US and other Western countries, where white people began to practice acupuncture in significant numbers, the model of delivery changed. In the US acupuncturists began to practice like psychotherapists or massage therapists: treating one patient per hour in individual rooms. Some US acupuncturists took their cue from Asian practitioners and would treat three or four patients an hour – but still used individual rooms. As US acupuncturists began treating patients individually, and fewer per hour, the cost of a single acupuncture treatment rose.

At the same time, the field professionalized. The first non-Asian acupuncturists were trained by Asian acupuncturists in informal settings and the training often took the form of an apprenticeship. A new generation of predominately white acupuncturists began to set up acupuncture schools, where the training took place in classrooms. Agencies were set up to accredit the schools and to administer a national certifying exam. Acupuncture schools offered federal student loans to their students. Acupuncturists made a conscious effort to model themselves after other, more established professionals such as chiropractors, physical therapists, osteopaths, and of course, medical doctors. Acupuncturists dreamed of being included in the health care mainstream, of receiving the kind of respect and compensation that other professionals received. Not surprisingly, the cost of acupuncture treatments and acupuncture education skyrocketed.

Unfortunately, however, utilization of acupuncture by ordinary consumers didn't keep pace, and neither did employment of acupuncturists. Estimates of how many people in the US receive acupuncture vary from 1% to 7%. Although some insurance plans cover acupuncture, most do not. Over 90% of acupuncturists are self-employed. Although data about professional attrition is hard to come by, it is generally accepted that about 75% of acupuncturists don't survive more than five years in practice, and most can't support themselves. The aspirations of the profession are lofty, but the economic reality on the ground is very, very grim.

Many acupuncturists and knowledgeable patients blame the underemployment of acupuncturists on mainstream health care's failure to accept and validate acupuncture. If only medical doctors respected acupuncture more, the logic goes, acupuncturists would be busy and everyone would be getting acupuncture. Doctors are hostile or skeptical, and that's why acupuncturists can't make a living. The solution then is for acupuncture education to include more biomedicine (and thus become longer and more expensive) so that acupuncturists can "talk" to doctors like peers.

Community acupuncturists don't buy this argument. Our experience is that most medical doctors are not hostile; most often they are neutral, and will encourage patients to use acupuncture if it helps. Many will refer patients if they have heard that other patients have gotten good results. And most doctors don't have any interest in talking to acupuncturists, because they're simply too busy. The problem with integrating acupuncture into American health care is not ideological, it's economic.

The economic infrastructure for acupuncture does not exist, for the most part, in Western countries, so patients don't use it, even if they and their doctors think it's a great idea. There are layers upon layers of economic disconnection. The cost of treatment is disconnected from what most patients of ordinary incomes can afford (between $75 -$300 for a single treatment). The cost of treatment is disconnected from the way acupuncture works best clinically. All the treatment protocols that US acupuncturists learned from Asia rely on courses of treatment, and a course of treatment can be anywhere from 10 to 100, delivered not less than a week apart, depending on the condition. Using one treatment when ten are called for is like taking one pill out of a course of antibiotics, and expecting it to work. Many insurance companies, even if they cover acupuncture, will not pay for a full course of treatment, and very few patients can afford to pay for it out of pocket. The consequence is that patients will save up so that they can get one treatment every six weeks or so – which is no help at all for any real health problem. The cost of acupuncture education is completely disconnected from what acupuncturists can expect to earn. The average student loan debt among graduates of one prominent acupuncture school was about $90,000 in 2009. Meanwhile the successful among them can expect to take home wages of $30,000 to $40,000 a year. Many can only afford to practice acupuncture on the side, as a hobby.

Perhaps the biggest disconnection is between the way acupuncture works and the for-profit nature of the American health care system. Profit is what usually pays for infrastructure. Acupuncture is too old to be patented, and so its use does not make investors any money. If acupuncture were a drug, it would be a wonder-drug, and the pharmaceutical company that held the patent for it would be richer than God. The list of conditions that acupuncture can relieve is very long, including asthma, arthritis, indigestion, PMS, sinusitis, insomnia, fibromyalgia, hot flashes, high blood pressure, infertility, constipation, anxiety, depression, the side effects of chemotherapy and the common cold, not to mention every conceivable variety of pain. All "side effects" are positive; it has stress reducing and mood elevating properties; furthermore, it is often so relaxing that many people who have nothing wrong with them use it on a regular basis, because they enjoy it so much. Yet it isn't addictive, and there's no way to overdose. Acupuncture is best suited to reducing medical costs for society, which could mean reducing the profit margins for certain parts of our health care system. Unfortunately, there is as yet little serious demand for acupuncture in America.

Given all these disconnections, you could reasonably claim that acupuncture exists as a profession in the US largely because acupuncture schools are able to offer federal student loans to their students, not because acupuncturists are busy treating many patients. What economic infrastructure there is for acupuncture is mostly borrowed: acupuncture as a profession has attached itself to the education industry. Acupuncture schools churn out hopeful students; students' tuition pays for acupuncture school accreditation; students pay exam fees, which supports a national certification agency; and licensed acupuncturists pay fees to the continuing education industry in order to keep up their certifications or in hopes of learning the secret that might allow them to finally make a living. With all these institutions doing business, there is the semblance of a profession. The problem is that the institutions are supported by people who are paying to *learn* acupuncture, while relatively few acupuncturists are adequately supported by people who are paying to *receive* acupuncture. In the last few decades, there's been a lot more learning of acupuncture than practicing of acupuncture, and the acupuncturists who do practice have not been organized.

There have always been a lot of different ways to practice acupuncture. Acupuncture is a very old, very human, thing. Humans have had at least two thousand years to do with it what they like to do with most things: practice it, adjust it, create variations on it, make up different schools of thought around it, and then in the face of all this interesting diversity, insist that their particular variation or school of thought is the only one that could possibly be correct. All the other variations and schools of thought are either ignorant, deluded, or outright harmful. In the case of acupuncture, there is absolutely no evidence that any variation or style of practice gets better clinical results than any other. The divisions between schools of thought and the arguments that arise as a result tend to keep acupuncturists from working together to address their economic problems.

Many acupuncturists in America have staked their entire identity on a particular style or school of practice. Their beliefs about acupuncture are more important to them and more substantial than anything else in their professional lives. They might have very few patients, or almost none; they might not be able to support themselves; they might have no supportive colleagues and no coworkers (because the practice of acupuncture is often terribly isolating). What they do have, however, is theories about acupuncture, and they hang on to those for dear life. The concrete, satisfying things that people usually get out of having a job – relationships, a good living, tangible results – can be in such short supply when you're an acupuncturist that, in order to preserve some self-esteem, you learn to focus on the abstract and tune out the concrete. For many acupuncturists, acupuncture is mostly an idea rather than a reality – including the idea of a career without the reality of a paycheck.

Acupuncture in the US is fundamentally out of context. It has become unmoored from the cultures that (probably) created it, and is mostly just floating, unrooted, in the West. If acupuncture were a plant, it would be a fragile epiphyte like an orchid: precariously attached to structures it didn't make, and living mostly on air. Despite all the potential good that acupuncture could do in American society, at this point, as far as most people are concerned, it's not a lot more useful than an orchid is. It's a lovely thing, but if we can't afford it – if acupuncturists can't afford to practice it, and patients can't afford to receive it – then all we can do is admire it at a distance. And what good is that, really?

My Personal Journey

This is where community acupuncture comes in, because community acupuncture has always been about trying to give acupuncture some meaningful, sustainable context.

I went to acupuncture school in 1991, soon after graduating from college. I had intended to go to medical school, but after a year volunteering full-time in an HIV service organization, I realized that I didn't like hospitals enough to spend more time in them. In the early 1990s, the antiretroviral drugs that effectively converted HIV from a death sentence into a manageable chronic illness had not yet been discovered. A lot of people with HIV were trying everything, including acupuncture. I was young and looking for a career; I didn't really understand the difference between going to acupuncture school and going to medical school. I thought both would prepare me for a career, and it was just a question of what kind of work I wanted to do after graduation. It never occurred to me that getting a degree in acupuncture was disconnected from getting work as an acupuncturist – that a Master's degree in acupuncture was more like a Master's degree in comparative literature than a medical degree. I didn't realize that I was going to a school that would teach me to *think* about something rather than to *do* something.

In 1994, I graduated from acupuncture school and the reality of my career choice began to set in. Relatively speaking, though, I was lucky. I got a part time job, and tried to start a private practice. My job was doing auricular acupuncture in a residential drug and alcohol treatment program. For this opportunity, I had NADA (National Acupuncture Detoxification Association)[4] to thank. One of their main goals is "to make acupuncture-based, barrier-free addiction

[4] http://www.acudetox.com/

treatment accessible to all communities and to ensure its integration with other treatment modalities." NADA uses a very simple protocol for ear acupuncture to treat drug addiction.[2] Ear acupuncture helps reduce drug cravings, insomnia, anxiety, and especially the acute misery of withdrawal from heroin and alcohol.

NADA is often closely associated with Alcoholics Anonymous and its related groups. In many treatment programs that use the NADA ear protocol, patients also attend twelve-step meetings. The idea is that an integral aspect of recovery from addiction is being part of a community. Generally, acupuncture sessions consist of patients sitting quietly together in a circle with ear needles for between 20 and 45 minutes, which reflects the structure of a twelve-step meeting, in which people in recovery come together in a group to share their process of healing.

In Spanish, NADA means "nothing," and the acronym was chosen on purpose. NADA is all about simplicity. The same five acupuncture points in the ears are used for every patient; the acupuncturist does not have to ask the patient any questions and the patient does not have to offer any information. To receive NADA style treatment, all the patient needs to do is clean their ears and sit down. A powerful shared stillness tends to arise from patients sitting together with ear needles. Many patients describe feeling deeply calm and centered while receiving acupuncture. Michael Smith, MD, one of the founders of NADA, sometimes describes this kind of treatment as "the hole in the doughnut": a place where patients can let go of all internal and external noise, a kind of nourishing emptiness which is rare and precious within the chaos of addiction. Creating a core of restful nothingness is useful for many problems besides addiction, and it's one of the things that acupuncture is really good at.

For seven years I was lucky enough to get a paycheck (albeit a small one) doing acupuncture in a variety of settings using the NADA[5] treatment protocol. Like many acupuncturists, I felt intimidated by the prospect of being self-employed, so I had a very small private practice to supplement my job. Fortunately, one of the clinics I worked at also had a "general medical acupuncture program." The clinic was a drug and alcohol treatment center that was mostly funded by the state and county; it provided housing, counseling, and other resources besides acupuncture to people in recovery. Most of its patients were chronically-homeless substance abusers. However, over the years, the "general medical program" had quietly and organically grown into a very modest income stream. Patients from the general public, not in the addictions treatment program, got acupuncture when it was being offered to the patients in the treatment program. These patients paid cash for acupuncture on a sliding scale from $5 to $30 per treatment, and included everyone from unemployed folks in public housing to a sympathetic state senator. As a result, I was able to gain experience treating a wide variety of conditions besides addiction and to interact with a wide range of patients. I learned that all kinds of ordinary people like to get acupuncture for all kinds of problems, as long as they can afford it.

When I attended acupuncture school in the early 1990s, the "going rate" for an acupuncture treatment was around $35; in 2013, it's anywhere from $75 - $300. I was in the unusual position of being able to compare the results of doing acupuncture with patients for whom payment was not an issue (the patients in the drug and alcohol program) or much less of an issue (the patients in the general medical clinic who

---

[5] NADA grew out of experiments in the South Bronx's Lincoln Hospital in the 1970s.

used a sliding scale) with patients for whom payment was a relentless, constant issue (the patients in my small private practice). Even though my private practice patients liked me and appreciated acupuncture, it was a struggle to get them to come in long enough, or often enough, for treatment. Acute problems are, in theory, best treated daily for several days, and I had the chance to see how effective that was at the public health clinic. However, because I was charging my private patients around $45 per treatment, it was unthinkable that they would come in every day for a week. The minute someone in my private practice began to get better, they would usually stop coming – even when I knew that the treatment wasn't really finished and their symptoms would soon return. By contrast, some of my sliding scale patients at the public health clinic came in regularly for months or years, often resulting in dramatic, though gradual, progress. Problems went away and stayed away. I felt I was seeing acupuncture as it was meant to be practiced.

Because the public health clinic that gave me this perspective was publicly funded, its continued existence was far from guaranteed. Over the years I survived several rounds of layoffs when county funding for health services was cut. I thought occasionally that it would be nice if the little stream of income from the sliding scale general medical patients could be grown into something that might pay for other services. The clinic's administration considered this as an "earned income strategy" similar to those that other nonprofits were exploring to stabilize funding, but in the end it came to nothing. The clinic was dependent on grants and government funding, and that was not going to change. This atmosphere of fiscal instability was stressful, and along with other stressors, it took its toll. After seven years I was burnt out, and beginning to wonder if I shouldn't take my chances in private practice, where if my work dried up it would be my own fault. When the inevitable next round of layoffs arrived, I volunteered.

Collecting unemployment and treating a few patients out of an extra room in my house gave me some needed time to think. Over a few months some general impressions began to coalesce into theories – which is a neat way of describing an internal process that was actually messy and confusing, and makes a lot more sense in hindsight than it did at the time. Without a job, I had to figure out how to make my private practice work; I loved doing acupuncture and I didn't really want to do anything else. After seven years, there was nothing else I was qualified to do.

I thought about why I was intimidated by the business of private practice, and realized that I was getting ready for another round of struggle with an issue that has appeared in some form at every important juncture in my life: class, and my feelings about it. Socioeconomic class in America is notoriously slippery, hard to define, and confusing. Many people deny its importance altogether. I know it matters because it's given me so much trouble.

What's Class Got To Do With It?

Until I was five I lived in South Baltimore, in the house my
great-grandparents bought when they got off the boat from
Germany. My father worked in a nearby chemical plant.
When I was old enough to go to school my parents moved
across the county line, because our nearest public school had a
reputation for violence, even in kindergarten, and I began a
lifelong process of colliding with invisible class boundaries.
Later on I would be able to explain that we had moved from a
working-class neighborhood to a lower middle-class
neighborhood; at the time what I knew was that my father
parked junk cars on the lawn, fixed everything with duct tape,
and the neighbors wanted us to go back where we came from.

Like many working-class families, my parents valued their
children's education, and being a smart kid who earned
scholarships, when the time came I went to the best college
that I could. That was Bryn Mawr, which besides having a
long Quaker tradition of concern for social justice, boasts some
lovely buildings contributed by the Rockefellers so that their
daughters would have a nice place to study. I have a vivid
memory of hearing a fellow student say that one of the things
she missed about being away from home was her cleaning
lady. "It's almost like she's part of the family," she explained. I
felt instantly and inexplicably queasy; it took me a while to
realize why – one of my aunts was somebody's cleaning lady.
My peers at college were the kind of people that my family
worked for. Where did I belong?

In acupuncture school I was taught that if I charged less than
the going rate in my private practice, I was acting as if
acupuncture and I weren't worth very much. Being an
impressionable student, for a while I actually believed it, but
of course at the same time I was aware on some level that this

meant that I was never going to be able to treat anybody like my own family.

It took me a long time to see what was obvious: as an acupuncturist, the only choices open to me at that time were to try to find patients who had enough disposable income to pay market rates for a course of treatment – upper middle-class patients – or to get a job in public health treating patients poor enough to qualify for the government to pay – which meant very poor indeed. There was no economic infrastructure in between – even though I knew very well from my own life that there were a vast number of potential patients in between.

Classism is generally defined as bias based on social or economic status. My personal definition for classism is the mechanism by which some people's lives are defined as less real or less valuable than others', based on their level of wealth, education, and culture. Looking at the structure of the acupuncture world at that time, people who had functional lives and modest resources did not exist as potential patients. They were completely invisible. If acupuncture clinics were restaurants, there would be only soup kitchens and four star bistros, with nothing in between. Since what would suit me best was something like a little neighborhood cafe, no wonder I had had trouble for years even contemplating private practice. Having figured this out, I realized that the existing economic structures of acupuncture were never going to work for me, or for any patient who was working-class, or for that matter, lower middle-class, or retired on a fixed income, or a student, or unemployed, or trying to put their kids through college. That's an awful lot of people. If I wanted to make my living as an acupuncturist, I was going to have to tear down all my assumptions, and everything I'd been taught, and start over. So I started to do that.

Once again, telling this in hindsight in neat paragraphs makes the process sound much more orderly and solitary than it actually was. In real life, I rented a commercial space in my working-class neighborhood, a few blocks from my house, and spent a lot of time moving furniture around until things looked right. The space, which I found myself weirdly in love with, was both improbably large and outrageously shabby by acupuncture standards. It had been a TV repair shop, and before that a print shop (not Monet kind of prints, but the heavy industry kind; the floor was reinforced in places with concrete so that the two-ton presses wouldn't fall through). When I first looked at it, it was a graveyard for second-hand furniture, some of which I bought. The rent was relatively low, the landlord was amazingly sympathetic, and I didn't know how I was going to afford it. But I had a lot of people helping me and I felt irrationally hopeful. I began to think about what working-class people consider important, and what they might value in an acupuncture clinic.

When I worked at the public health clinic with the sliding scale acupuncture program, periodically I would encourage my working-class neighbors who needed acupuncture to go there – since they couldn't afford my private-practice fees. Not one of them ever went. They had various excuses: they didn't want to drive downtown, the hours were inconvenient, whatever was hurting them didn't hurt that bad anyway. Over time I suspected the truth: they knew that the clinic was located in a treatment program that mostly served homeless people, which made it automatically off-limits. Not that my neighbors had anything against homeless people – some of them volunteered in their churches' soup kitchens – but it was unthinkable that they, being working-class, should in any way be on the receiving end of charity. They would not go to a nonprofit clinic for poor people, unless they went as helpers themselves.

If I was going to get them into my clinic, nothing about it could feel like I was trying to "help the needy." Which, fortunately, I wasn't; I was trying to make a living treating patients I could relate to, but nonetheless there was a lot of mental furniture to discard. First to go was the practice that people either paid the market rate for treatment ($65, in 2002) or proved that they deserved a reduced fee by bringing in tax returns or bank statements – which is what other acupuncturists did. For years I had assumed that there was no other way to have someone pay less than the market rate, but as I swept out my cavernous, industrial new space and thought my rebellious new thoughts, this suddenly looked like a humiliating, ridiculous bit of institutional classism. Nobody in my neighborhood could pay $65. I already knew that. Why should they have to prove it? Anyway, who said that acupuncture should cost $65 per treatment in the first place? Not the Yellow Emperor's Classic of Internal Medicine, that's for sure. This was my clinic and I could set my fees however I wanted to. I knew I wanted to use a sliding scale, because I had seen it translate into accessibility for a wide range of people. I would use a sliding scale, but people could choose an amount within the range based on what they felt comfortable with, no justification required. This would be acupuncture as an affordable, local business instead of a charity. I knew my neighbors would support that.

I realized I was going to have a hard time creating a conventional-looking acupuncture clinic out of my cobwebby, cement-floored new digs; maybe I shouldn't even try. The patients I wanted, not having ever had acupuncture, wouldn't be expecting it anyway. A lot of my neighbors would be actively uncomfortable in the upscale ambience of most conventional acupuncture clinics, and if I was going to ask them to come in every day or every week for treatment, I couldn't make them uncomfortable.

Thinking about their comfort led to thinking about the issue of professional demeanor, which is relentlessly preached in acupuncture schools. But what if acting like a doctor was just an excuse for charging doctor's fees? I realized that *I* didn't like being on the receiving end of a professional demeanor; it made me feel subtly ashamed. If I had a problem, I wanted to feel that the person helping me was competent, kind, and above all, understood me. A conventional acupuncturist probably wouldn't understand what it's like to be working-class. I decided to try really hard not to talk down to my patients, and not to sound like an acupuncturist.

By this time I had been in practice long enough to know what most clinicians know, which is that when it comes to garden-variety problems such as headaches, bad digestion, or back pain – the bulk of what most acupuncturists treat – the resolution of the problem usually involves some common sense. In fact, most patients know deep down what to do to get better; for some reason or another they just aren't doing it. They know they get a headache when they spend too much time with certain people, or get constipated when they don't eat properly, or have back spasms when they work too hard. Acupuncture excels at relieving pain, but to really deal with the root of the problem, you usually have to find a way to get the patients to listen to themselves. What if I set up my clinic with the view that I wanted a place where people could listen to themselves, rather than having to listen to me lecturing them?

Many upper middle-class patients are perfectly comfortable paying professionals for copious personal attention. Some of them like it the way they like shopping; a personal relationship with a "healing professional" is just one more thing to buy. Working-class people by and large are not like this; many aren't used to being fussed over, and they don't like it. I already knew my neighbors well enough to know that if they were going to include acupuncture in their already busy, complex lives, coming to the clinic would have to be easy. I couldn't require them to put a lot of energy into their relationship. In fact, they didn't necessarily want me to act like their best friend or their therapist. They would want their problems to be resolved, with as little attendant drama as possible. It would be best if my professional presence took a back seat to the acupuncture. The way the clinic worked would have to be simple. Working-class people tend to like simplicity, or maybe they just need it; when you are working two jobs and raising a family, you don't really have room for unnecessary complexity and posturing from your acupuncturist.

Opening Shop

It was clear that I was moving toward something like NADA treatment. And yet, I didn't want to focus on treating addiction; I had seen enough to believe that treating addiction with acupuncture alone, without counseling, housing or job training, was not adequate. But what if treating people very simply, in a community setting, didn't have to be all about addictions or ear acupuncture? Why not treat back pain or headaches or arthritis in a group? Why should group treatment even have to happen in a group? Why try to get everyone to come at the same time and have the same treatment?

Treating back pain with acupuncture does not require sticking needles in the back. In fact, there are several schools of acupuncture that suggest putting needles in the places that hurt is a bad idea, and that points in the hand or the ankle work better for back pain than points in the back. I had experimented with these treatment strategies and found them effective. Supposing I didn't need to have anyone lay down? What if I could treat everyone in chairs?

I found twelve second-hand recliners and arranged them in groups of three or four in one of my big rooms. I added some rugs, some lamps, and some plants. It looked like the living room of somebody who had a very large family. I could imagine my neighbors sitting in these chairs, relaxing with needles in their hands and feet and head. I knew how to treat most problems using only needles in the hands, feet, and head; nobody would have to take their clothes off. If I didn't spend a lot of time lecturing, pretending to be a doctor, I could treat four to six patients an hour. They wouldn't have to come in at the same time; I could schedule appointments every ten or fifteen minutes. Patients who were nervous about acupuncture could come in with family or friends and watch other people having a good experience. Couples could come in together; parents could bring their kids. Working-class people tend to take it for granted that relationships, family, and community are a good thing; I thought they would accept being treated together as a natural event.

When I began working in public health as an acupuncturist, my pay was $15 an hour. The going rate in 2002 for a 1-hour private treatment was $65 an hour. So if instead of treating one person per hour for $65, could I create a sliding scale of $15 to $35 per treatment and treat four to six people an hour? If so, I could earn between $60 to $210 per hour. And, as important, I'd make acupuncture available to up to six people, instead of just one. Even if only one person showed up in an hour and paid me $15, it would be like having a job again! In this way, I could value community –my community, in which nobody was going to pay me $65 per treatment but most people could afford at least $15 – and not lose money. Maybe I'd even make a living. That was the extent of my financial planning.

Making acupuncture affordable by thinking in terms of a community of patients led to realizing that, if I were successful, I could avoid any financial entanglements with anything outside of that little community. I wouldn't need to bill insurance, since my fees would be comparable to most co-pays. I wouldn't need to seek grants or government funding – which I really didn't want to do, having had plenty of time to appreciate what an unstable financial base those were. (By the time I was making these calculations, most of my public health co-workers who were acupuncturists no longer had jobs.) This supported another working-class value, which is independence; families and communities taking care of each other is valued and important, but being taken care of by any big outside entity like a corporation or the government is often frowned upon.

After all the furniture moving, the contemplation, and after my partner Skip and our kids painted the walls over a long weekend, what we ended up with was:

- a big central room with 12 recliners as the main clinic space; nothing fancy, yet comfortable, soft, and soothing;
- a sliding scale of $15 to $35 per treatment, based on the patient's assessment of what they could comfortably afford;
- an appointment book with appointments every 10 minutes; and
- a set of principles for my new business that I christened "Working Class Acupuncture."

Working Class Acupuncture (WCA) would not be about charity; it would be a low-cost, high-volume business plan for a sustainable community business. Patients who couldn't afford to pay market rates for acupuncture are not necessarily suffering from "financial hardship," and scholarships or individually reduced rates are not a solution. The point would be to lower the barriers, not to make a few exceptions to the upper middle-class rule. Acupuncture treatments should be simple, frequent, and regular – that is how they are most effective. What makes acupuncture work is the patient's energy, and the clinic setup should reflect this: a welcoming atmosphere, minimal use of tables, no white coats and no professional posturing. It's good to have a lot of patients receiving acupuncture in the same space at the same time: it's not an absence of privacy, it's the presence of a collective energetic field that makes treatments more powerful. Healing is not an elitist commodity, and it shouldn't be any big deal.

Everybody who knew anything about acupuncture was skeptical, at best. We were told that there was no market and that affordable acupuncture clinics don't grow. We were told that working-class patients don't want acupuncture, because they're not educated or sophisticated enough to appreciate it, and that they don't value their health; they spend all their money on beer, cigarettes, and cable TV. We were told that anybody who was willing to try acupuncture would never be willing to try it in a group. We were told that our sliding scale was illegal (it's not). We were told that we were breaking laws by treating people in groups (we're not). We were told that we were devaluing the profession with our low prices and our second-hand recliners. And finally, when we got mad, we were told that we shouldn't be angry because it wasn't spiritual and acupuncturists were supposed to be spiritual; we should try to be more friendly to all of the acupuncturists who were suggesting that our mere existence was making them look bad, and could we please stop?

We didn't. We made a lot of mistakes, but our affordable acupuncture clinic did grow. Skip was able to leave his public health job and came on staff. By 2006, when I wrote the original *Remedy*, we had employees and we were giving about 200 treatments a week. In 2013, we have three locations and we're giving about 900 treatments per week. The original principles of operation remain basically the same, because they proved so effective – not only could I make a modest living (and a few other acupuncturists could too), but people in my community could afford to come in for acupuncture often enough to get better, some of them dramatically so. It worked beautifully, and naturally, to create a steady cash flow from many small sources, rather than trying to tap a single big pipe of insurance or government funding.

I was delighted; I could do what I loved without abandoning the people with whom I identified. I had figured out where I belonged. Even better, a lovely consequence of the sliding scale was that people from all kinds of backgrounds came to the clinic and ended up relaxing together in the same room. Class divisions melted down every day into a cozy sea of sleeping patients. People told us constantly how much they appreciated it. I felt like I had won my own private class war.

But... only if I defined victory very, very narrowly. One day, my college friend Laura, living in New Jersey, called to tell me that she was pregnant, and asked if acupuncture could help with her morning sickness. "Of course," I said. She called back a week later, thrilled; she had seen an acupuncturist and was feeling much better. How wonderful that this was what I was doing with my life! "Thanks, Laura," I said, "I'm so glad to hear that, and it would be really good for both you and the baby if you could go back every week throughout your pregnancy." There was dead silence on the other end of the phone for a moment. "Lisa, the treatment cost $175. I can't go back."

Of course this phenomenon wasn't limited to my friends. One of my patients had a sister in Florida who was going through chemotherapy, and she knew acupuncture would help with the nausea and the stress. There are a lot of acupuncturists in Florida, but since her sister earns $9 an hour as a preschool teacher, there was no one she could afford. Patients were enthusiastic about acupuncture and wanted to share it with their extended families and friends, but unless they lived in Portland, it was financially out of the question. Often they got excited enough that they would call acupuncturists to set up appointments – and only then find out that it was out of their reach. It seemed cruel to get people's hopes up, especially when what they were hoping for was relief from pain. I realized that when patients asked me about referrals, what I was really saying was "Sorry, acupuncture is not for the likes of you, unless you can find an anomaly like us."

At the same time I became aware that we were also an anomaly from another perspective: we were a couple of acupuncturists (in Portland, a city supposedly oversaturated with acupuncturists) who were able to make our living solely doing acupuncture. We were paying our mortgage; we were feeding our kids. A colleague who spoke with acupuncturists around the country as part of his business told me that he estimated that most acupuncturists were seeing an average of twelve patients a week, and that maybe a quarter of all licensed acupuncturists were working full time at their practice. I pictured my friend in New Jersey and my patient's sister in Florida surrounded by frustrated acupuncturists working at Starbucks. I wondered if we could do something about the larger problem. I didn't necessarily want a lot of other acupuncturists calling themselves Working Class Acupuncture – because I knew from experience that there weren't very many acupuncturists with working-class backgrounds – so I began to write more generally about a low-cost, high volume business designed to make acupuncture accessible to people with ordinary incomes, and I referred to it as "community acupuncture."[6]

---

[6] I can't remember exactly who came up with this term. It might have been Mary Saunders in Boulder, who opened the second clinic using the model.

Yes, We CAN

By 2006, it was clear that there was a lot of interest in community acupuncture. Skip and I put out a zine that we titled, *The Little Red Book of Working Class Acupuncture*, since by then we'd been accused by other acupuncturists of being communists. We mailed it to about 100 acupuncturists for $5 apiece. I was writing regular columns on social entrepreneurship for an industry newspaper, *Acupuncture Today*, and since there were not very many examples of social entrepreneurship in acupuncture, the columns were all about community acupuncture. Their website had online comment forums for columnists. The other columnists' comment forums were gathering cobwebs and spam, but mine was full of lively conversation. That gig lasted from 2005 to early 2007, when the paper fired me because they felt my ideas had "dangerous potential" for the acupuncture profession. (I can only assume that nobody on their staff had been reading the columns until 2007. The editor who had hired me disappeared at the same time as my column.)

By that time we had gotten together with a sympathetic (and disillusioned) executive director of one of the professional acupuncture organizations, and he had helped us set up a new 501(c)(6) nonprofit, the Community Acupuncture Network (CAN).[7] It had its own website with forums – and not a minute too soon, because other people were opening up community acupuncture clinics and wanting to talk about it. In October 2006 we put on our first workshop, and by the end of that year we were signing up members; we had our own professional association, and with *The Remedy*, we had a book that was almost, but not quite, a manual.

---

[7] Many thanks to Michael R. McCoy, Ph.D. The other founding Board members of CAN were Lupine Hudson of WCA and me.

CAN was my first experience of camaraderie with other acupuncturists. Apart from NADA, CAN was the only acupuncture organization concerned about social justice. Perhaps as a result, a lively spirit of self-help emerged among us. Many acupuncturists, in addition to being isolated, tend to be competitive and secretive. Since so few people get acupuncture, there's often a sense of patient scarcity. We were trying to reach a vast, underserved patient base, so we didn't need to be territorial. CAN made a conscious effort to get acupuncturists to share experiences, knowledge, and encouragement, and so it often felt like a big online support group. The gaps in *The Remedy* about how to create a community acupuncture clinic got filled in from conversations on the website. It was a first stab at a collective approach – a radical departure from business as usual in the acupuncture profession. Acupuncture organizations often struggle to cultivate enthusiasm among their members, but for us it was easy. When it became clear that patients were referring their out of town family and friends to other CAN clinics, we knew we were on the right track.

We also knew that we had no clue about building a nonprofit organization, and lots of things about CAN, couldn't. Yet. But it was effective at inspiring other acupuncturists to ignore what they had been taught in school about low prices devaluing the profession. There was a lot of pent-up demand for an alternative to the conventional low-volume, high-cost, white-coat approach. With a whole group of people pursuing the same experiment, we began to refer to "the community acupuncture model" or just "the model." CAN gave all of us a big laboratory. Acupuncturists all over the country were trying out the model, testing variations and approaches, and because we were all connected online and talking (constantly) about the results, it became an effective open-source community.

We began to get media attention. The first time a writer referred to "the community acupuncture movement" it seemed like a joke. The second time, we didn't laugh so quickly. After a while, we began to use the term ourselves. It was clear, after all, that *something* was moving.[8]

---

[8] For example: http://postgrowth.org/community-acupuncture-a-non-consumptive-healthcare-model/

Community Acupuncture Defined

So what is Community Acupuncture really? We define it as the practice of offering acupuncture:

1) in a setting where multiple patients receive treatments at the same time;

2) by financially sustainable and accountable means;

3) within a context of accessibility created by consistent hours, frequent treatments, affordable services, and lowering all the barriers to treatment that we possibly can, for as many people as possible, while continuing to be financially self-sustaining; and

4) with a commitment to social justice in health care.

Acupuncture Theories In Context

One of the things that we talked about a lot within CAN was acupuncture theories: what worked and how, and which theories fit the community acupuncture model.

At the same time I was opening WCA, I was having an experience that would cause me to question the role of acupuncture theories in real-life acupuncture practice. I was getting the acupuncture education that I didn't get in acupuncture school, and my teachers were a couple named Bobette and Harry (nicknamed Chico) Senn.

The Senns had had the kind of life that people write memoirs about. They met in Southern California when Chico had a well-paying corporate job and volunteered in local Republican politics. They lived a Southern California Republican lifestyle until they gave it all up and moved to Mist, Oregon, to make furniture for a living and raise their children in the woods. They had a large and colorful cast of friends: artisans who sold their wares at Portland Saturday market, some of the people who run Oregon's annual Country Fair, and people who went to their church. Lots of different kinds of people enjoyed Bobette and Chico for their warmth, their wit, and their creativity. When I met them, they were living in a charming old house in Portland. Bobette was a seamstress, and Chico was dying of lung cancer. I was working for Kaiser Hospice on a pilot project, treating hospice patients for anxiety. I met the Senns in 1999, and this is their story:

My name is Bobette Senn. My husband, Chico, was diagnosed with metastatic lung cancer in 1993. He had surgery and radiation, and responded pretty well, but by 1999 he was on hospice. We were introduced to acupuncture because at that time Kaiser Hospice offered five in-home acupuncture treatments to patient and caregiver. I wanted to try it, but Chico was reluctant. He did it for me, because I couldn't get it unless he got it too. Once he tried it, he liked it very much. He was looking for anything positive he could find, to help him keep fighting, and it made him feel better. We looked forward to the acupuncturist coming every week.

When the five treatments were up, Chico wanted to keep getting acupuncture, and the hospice nurses found a facility that would continue the treatments on a sliding-fee scale. Otherwise we could never have afforded it; we were on OHP and Medicare. Chico wanted to reduce the amount of morphine he was taking, partly because the Medicare laws had changed and it had gotten really expensive for us.

We got acupuncture once a week for three years, and then twice a week for two more years. As a result of getting acupuncture once a week, he got off Oxycodone completely, and reduced his total narcotic use by 70%. He gradually got better; he started mowing the lawn, trimming the hedges, playing golf. We traveled, and he didn't get a wheelchair at the airport, he would walk. He gradually came back to living a fairly normal life. He would get winded, of course. But he went fishing. He babysat our grandson. We would leave acupuncture and go do errands all day. His health would always get worse in the winter, but acupuncture would pull him through.

Each time he got a treatment, it would give him the energy to go until the next treatment. It sustained him. It calmed him. It gave him the will to continue to fight.

It added five years to his life.

When we started getting acupuncture twice a week, his energy really progressed, and he started doing something he hadn't done in a long time, which was playing music. Chico was a drummer. He played with some famous jazz musicians when he was younger. He loved to play. Music was a big part of his life. It was so good for him. I can't tell you how much enjoyment he got out of it. He would say that *when he played, he felt 17 and not 70.*

Chico always used visualization, and he prayed constantly. Acupuncture worked along with all of the faith that he had. Acupuncture was a piece of the puzzle that made up the whole picture – along with prayer and visualization and music – the whole picture of five more years of living together, of being happy, and without acupuncture, that picture would not have been there.

As far as being the caregiver, acupuncture gave me a calmness – not just because of the treatments themselves, but in knowing that Chico was doing something for himself. It was something we shared together. I'm going to keep doing acupuncture because it gives me energy and I know it's preventing bigger health problems. I don't want to take pills for every little thing. I want to be able to control my own health with any alternative that's reasonable to me. (From The Little Red Book of Working Class Acupuncture, 10th Anniversary Edition)

I started treating Chico and Bobette at their house, and then at the public health facility with the sliding-scale general medicine program where I worked. After I was laid off, I treated them at my house, and finally at WCA. Part of the pressure I felt to provide affordable acupuncture came not just from my own working-class background and loyalties, but from my present-day relationship with Chico and Bobette. Like a lot of other people who knew them, I found them irresistible, and also, something significant seemed to be happening with the treatments. When Chico got regular acupuncture, he stopped coughing up blood and his energy was good. If he missed a treatment, he started coughing up blood again and his energy declined. I had reason to think that for Chico, getting acupuncture was very possibly a matter of life and death.

The thing about treating Chico though, was that he hated

needles. He really, really hated them. I used very thin needles, and put them in very gently, and he could barely stand it. He couldn't tolerate being treated the way I was used to treating people, and this is how my acupuncture education, or re-education, began.

There's a famous acupuncture book titled *The Web That Has No Weaver*. It's the book that taught many Americans how to think about acupuncture. Here's a quote from the Forward, written in 1983: "Although acupuncture itself has gained some acceptance, the Western medical and scientific community has never considered seriously the medical tradition and culture from which the technique sprang. As if a full understanding of acupuncture were encompassed by knowing where to stick the needles!"

As if! (As they say in Southern California).

The Web That Has No Weaver goes on to lay out, in 400 pages, the theoretical framework of what is known as Traditional Chinese Medicine (TCM). The logic that forms the foundation of TCM is the same that informs Chinese philosophy and Chinese cosmology. Its most basic aspect is Yin-Yang theory, or the idea that everything in the universe depends on a balance of complementary opposites. In this passage, the author compares a Chinese physician to a Chinese landscape painter:

"...the Chinese think of each person as a cosmos in miniature. A person manifests the same patterns as does the painting or the universe. The Yang or Fire aspects of the body are the dynamic or transforming, while the Yin or Water aspects are the more yielding and nourishing... Harmony and health are the balanced interplay of these tendencies. In each person, as in every landscape, there are signs that, when balanced, define health or beauty. If the signs are out of balance, the person is ill or the painting is ugly. So the

Chinese physician looks at a patient the way a painter looks at a landscape – as a particular arrangement of signs in which the essence of the whole can be seen...This artistic sensitivity allows the physician to stay in touch with subtle refinements of meaning...Chinese medicine is not primarily quantitative. It recognizes that each person's pattern has a unique texture; each image has an essential quality." (From *The Web That Has No Weaver*, pg 18-19)

In school, I was taught that the most important part of my job was to accurately diagnose the most subtle aspects of how each individual patient was out of balance. Correct diagnosis actually mattered more than treating the person with acupuncture. With correct diagnosis, an acupuncturist could prescribe Chinese herbs and teach a person how to change their lifestyle so that they could come back into balance and be healthy. All of this was infinitely more important than just "where to stick the needles"; this delicate, precise diagnosis is the pride of an acupuncturist. The only problem was, Chico was having none of it.

I had learned a particular method of Japanese pulse diagnosis in school that I really liked: I read the patient's pulse, and a kind of Yin-Yang formula told me which points I should needle. The most important ones were on the hands and feet; they were the linchpin of the entire treatment. Chico wouldn't let me needle his hands or his feet. I couldn't needle his back, either, because he'd had so much radiation that his ribs in the back had broken, and he didn't want to be needled there (where some of the most powerful acupuncture points were supposed to be). He would let me needle his chest, and his elbows, and sometimes his knees – as long as I did it very carefully and shallowly. The acupuncture treatments I did on Chico would never have been approved by my supervisors in my school's student clinic, because from the perspective of any Traditional Chinese Medical theory, the needles were too few, too shallow, and in the wrong places.

As *The Web That Has No Weaver* points out, and many acupuncturists are eager to tell you, there is so much more to Traditional Chinese Medicine than just acupuncture. Take Chinese herbs! But Chico didn't want to take Chinese herbs, and couldn't have afforded them if he did. Then there's lifestyle counseling, talking about Chinese medical nutrition and practices like qi gong, something we were encouraged to spend a lot of time on with patients in the student clinic. Chico was an evangelical Christian who read his Bible while he got acupuncture; he was happy with his spiritual practices and wasn't interested in learning any new ones. And nutrition! All first year acupuncture students learn that the worst possible food for any illness, from a TCM perspective, is ice cream; Chico drank a milkshake every single day. He felt that it was good for him.

One day in 2002, not long after opening WCA, the phone rang. It was Chico's doctor, who was also the head of pulmonology at the local Kaiser hospital. I was surprised, because by then I had learned that, contrary to what I was taught in school, doctors don't want to talk to acupuncturists – they don't have time. Chico's doctor wanted to talk about his yearly chest X-ray, which was the only diagnostic test that Chico got anymore. Even though Chico had officially been kicked out of hospice a couple of years ago, neither Chico nor his doctor was going to try to treat his cancer aggressively, so there was no point in doing a lot of tests. His doctor told me that the X-ray showed that the cancer had stopped growing. It hadn't moved in a year. He wanted to know if I had an explanation, since the only change in Chico's treatment was that he was getting a lot of acupuncture, and presumably I knew what was going on. But I didn't know what was going on, other than that everything I had been taught about how to do acupuncture was apparently wrong. I didn't say that to the pulmonologist, of course; I just told him I didn't know, either. There was a silence on the other end of the phone. "OK," he said, "In that case, I have a request. Can you do something about getting him off the morphine? If his cancer isn't progressing, I can't justify continuing to prescribe so much morphine." I said I would try, and hung up the phone, stunned.

Acupuncture wasn't a cure, of course. Chico passed away in 2004. But looking back to all that had happened since I met him in 1999, I had to agree with Bobette that the treatment had apparently added five years to his life.

Every acupuncturist who has been in practice for any amount of time can recall treatments that didn't work. Often these treatments are memorable because of how hard the acupuncturist was trying to come up with the perfect treatment, how careful the diagnosis was, how much research went into choosing the points – and still, the treatment didn't help the patient. You did everything right, but it didn't matter. With treating Chico, I was discovering the corollary that all longtime acupuncturists also know: sometimes the treatments where you did everything wrong got the most spectacular results. A decade of that kind of thing is enough to make you skeptical about "right" and "wrong."

I had been an acupuncturist long enough to know there were different schools of acupuncture theory. All of them could claim about the same degree of clinical success – though I didn't know anybody else whose patient had gotten kicked out of hospice as a result of acupuncture. Acupuncture worked, no matter how you explained it. And it worked when you didn't bother to explain it. "Just sticking needles in" was, as far as I could tell, more important than doing a TCM diagnosis. As a result of treating Chico, my faith in Chinese medical theories was shot to hell, and at the same time, I felt newly determined to do whatever it took to make acupuncture available to anybody who wanted to try it. How many more people like Chico were out there? If I had reason to believe that acupuncture, stripped down to its bare essentials, really could add five years to somebody's life – and I did, I had seen it – didn't I have an obligation to reorganize my professional priorities? Maybe other acupuncturists' disdain for "just sticking needles in" wasn't enough reason not to promote it, if it could do for even one other person what it had apparently done for Chico.

This proved hard to explain to other acupuncturists, and to some patients as well.

A lot of people love acupuncture precisely because its theories are beautiful. Thinking about how the elements in a Chinese landscape painting relate to the elements in the human body is a lot more refined and pleasant than thinking about somebody coughing up blood, and what you might be obligated to do about it. The delicate balance of yin and yang is a more appealing thing to contemplate than the gross social inequities that make it hard for someone to afford pain medication. It's understandable that most acupuncturists would choose to pay attention to the former, not the latter. But I just couldn't anymore. With Chico I had seen what acupuncture could do when it was a reality and not just an idea. Reality had reached out and grabbed me, and it wouldn't let go; it kept demanding that I shed all the ideas I'd learned in school that didn't match.

Acupuncture isn't rocket science, and it isn't mysticism. It's possible to approach it in a very simple, practical way. I still use some kinds of diagnosis in my practice, but they're the most streamlined, and least time-consuming. The reality is that many patients don't really need a diagnosis. The "side effects" of acupuncture treatments are increased energy, better sleep, improvement in mood, and reduction in stress. You can memorize point protocols and just stick the needles in, and people get the relief that they're looking for. This is dangerous heresy from the point of view of the acupuncture profession, but it's true. If you're treating enough patients, you can prove it, over and over again.

A lot of patients love acupuncture because the process of diagnosis makes them feel "like a cosmos in miniature" with their own unique pattern. It's interesting to have an acupuncturist take your pulse and tell you that your Liver is constrained, or your Yin is deficient, or your Yang is rising. Most people like to learn things about themselves, and a TCM diagnosis can feel like a special, private kind of knowledge, a portrait of yourself in Chinese calligraphy. There's nothing inherently wrong with that, but how it plays out in real life can be problematic, when it's taken out of context.

There is no evidence that acupuncture using this kind of diagnosis gets better clinical results than acupuncture that doesn't. There's plenty of anecdotal evidence that what acupuncturists are thinking about when they put the needles in has little to do with what happens in the body afterwards. As a therapy, acupuncture is like a shotgun, not a laser. It's very common for patients to tell acupuncturists that conditions and symptoms have improved with treatment when the acupuncturist didn't even know about those conditions or symptoms, because the patient was being treated for something else altogether. As an acupuncturist, you can only aim your treatment to a certain degree; the effects of what you do are still going to go all over the place. So it's not entirely honest to give patients the impression that a precise diagnosis is always the key to good clinical results, because it just isn't.

Stressing a TCM diagnosis can also pathologize a patient's experience and make them, well, stressed. I've had plenty of patients tell me, with real anxiety, that their last acupuncturist told them that their Liver and Kidneys were weak. Having stagnant Liver qi is the norm if you live in a Western culture. Having deficient kidney Yin and Yang as you age is to be expected. If you're an average middle-aged person living in America, from a TCM perspective, your Liver and Kidneys are probably weak, relative to an average teenager living in a more relaxed culture. Certainly you can choose to get acupuncture, and you'll probably feel better. But giving a patient a diagnosis, in our society, is a way of hooking them into the medical system and making them think that they need treatment.

It's one thing to offer people acupuncture in the hope that it benefits them; it's quite another to scare them into getting it. I've heard stories of famous Chinese acupuncturists who felt a patient's pulse and sent them straight to the hospital, where the cancer that their MD had missed was promptly diagnosed. But I've also heard of acupuncturists who build their businesses by doing pulse readings at health fairs, and tell prospective patients that if they really love their children, they'll "invest in their health" with a series of expensive acupuncture treatments to address their imbalances. If those imbalances aren't addressed, they'll surely get worse and worse – this is what ancient Chinese wisdom tells us – and don't you want to see your children grow up? There are a lot more people with diagnosable TCM patterns that don't need treatment – everybody has some "imbalance" in their pulses – than there are people with hidden cancers that only a TCM master can diagnose.

Our society is suffering from isolation and alienation, in part because we value individualism so much. It's necessary to look at how acupuncture in our culture either fits that paradigm, or helps heal it. Giving every patient an elaborate TCM diagnosis, regardless of whether or not they're really ill, contributes to a hyper-individualized approach to acupuncture, and ignores the social context. Acupuncture claims to be holistic, but how holistic is it to teach patients to focus narrowly on their own individual symptoms, and tune out the rest of society? Acupuncture doesn't have to just be about what *my* acupuncturist felt in *my* pulses, and what she told me I had to eat for breakfast from now on. Acupuncture can be about pain relief and stress relief on a big scale, for hundreds of thousands of people who need it. Acupuncture can be about inclusion: being glad that your neighbors are having a better quality of life because they're getting treatments that they can afford. Whether we prioritize the individual or the collective when we do acupuncture is entirely our choice. Community acupuncturists believe that the individual gets prioritized plenty in our society already, and one way of bringing balance to the situation is to use acupuncture collectively, to bring the greatest benefit to the greatest number of patients.

Social Business

By 2007, we had a term for what we were doing with the community acupuncture model: "social business." Muhammad Yunus, the 2006 Nobel Peace Prize winner, coined the term to describe "a non-loss, non-dividend company that is cause-driven rather than profit-driven, with the potential to act as a change agent for the world" (*Creating a World without Poverty: Social Business and the Future of Capitalism,*" pg 22.)

From the start, WCA was a social business – a business designed to provide social dividends to the larger community as opposed to financial profits to individual owners or shareholders. The social dividends of our business were affordable treatments for residents of a working-class neighborhood, and a livable wage for the acupuncturists providing the treatments, who lived in the neighborhood. Our business had two major demands to balance: the need to keep the treatments affordable for our neighbors, and the need for us to support our household (without having to take on second jobs). We were successful at meeting those two demands, but we were not successful in generating profits beyond that. We broke even, no more; but we broke even *reliably.* As we hired more acupuncturists and treated more patients, we kept breaking even. Our patient numbers were more consistent than any other acupuncture practice we'd ever heard of, and some of our patients became passionate advocates of affordable acupuncture. They supported us in all kinds of ways we never expected: they built bike racks for us, got a story about our clinic on a local TV program, tracked down used recliners (and often delivered them), and handed out our cards by the dozen while cashiering at the grocery store. We were treating people who never imagined they'd be able to get acupuncture; we were connecting with people we never thought we'd be able to connect with. We knew nothing about business and had no real idea what we were doing, but it was thrilling. It was nice to know what to call it.

One of Muhammad Yunus' central arguments for social business is that capitalism, according to economic theory, makes human beings one-dimensional, motivated only by personal economic gain. The desire to maximize individual profits is far from the only force that moves people. In real life, people are much more complex; they are genuinely interested in solving social and environmental problems for their own sake; they care about their neighbors because it feels good to care about one's neighbors. Selflessness is real and under the right circumstances, it can have real power.

We can testify to the truth of this. A number of acupuncturists told us that people who wanted acupuncture would never accept our delivery method. The entire point of alternative medicine in America, they told us, was that individuals could get maximum individual attention from a health care professional wearing a white coat. Nobody who had experienced conventional acupuncture and liked it would ever want to get treated in a shabby industrial space surrounded by – horrors – people who obviously didn't have much money. When one acupuncturist saw our logo, a red fist with stars where the acupuncture points of the Heart meridian are, he said, "It looks like you're inviting people to a revolution. People don't want that; they want to be pampered." It turns out that Muhammad Yunus was right and he was wrong. People are more complicated than that.

Certainly WCA was not everybody's cup of tea. As we expected, many of our patients had never had acupuncture before because they couldn't afford it; once they had tried it, some of them wanted more of it, and some of them didn't. There was an entirely different demographic, however, that had had acupuncture before, and were delighted with WCA nonetheless. Plenty of people who had had expensive, one-on-one, private room acupuncture thought it was really cool that not only could they now get as much acupuncture as they wanted, but that lots of people they didn't know, people of different backgrounds and ages and races, could get it too. Certainly, some patients just tolerated the ancient recliners and the DIY vibe in order to get acupuncture that they couldn't afford elsewhere; but some patients loved it, loved it all, without reservation. If having acupuncture in a room with a lot of other people meant that their grandmothers and aunties on fixed incomes (everybody seemed to have an aunty on a fixed income) could get it too, then forget about the individual attention and the white coat. Bring on the community! Patients all over the country in CAN clinics were proving that their concerns didn't stop at the boundaries of their own skin. It really mattered to them that other people could get acupuncture; it made them feel good about getting treated in community clinics.

Quotations from Muhammad Yunus

"We have to get out of this mindset that the rich will do the business and the poor will have the charity."

Clinton Global Initiative, September 20, 2011

"I am proposing to create another kind of business, based on selflessness that is in all of us. I am calling it social business."

Nelson Mandela Annual Lecture, July 11, 2009

"I should never seek a job in my life, my mission in life is to create jobs. I am not a job seeker, I am a job giver."

Nelson Mandela Annual Lecture, July 11, 2009

"The challenge I set before anyone who condemns private-sector business is this: If you are a socially conscious person, why don't you run your business in a way that will help achieve social objectives?"

— Muhammad Yunus, Banker To The Poor: Micro-Lending and the Battle Against World Poverty

"I profoundly believe, as Grameen's experience over twenty years has shown, that personal gain is not the only possible fuel for free enterprise. Social goals can replace greed as a powerful motivational force. Social-consciousness-driven enterprises can be formidable competitors for the greed-based enterprises. I believe that if we play our cards right, social-consciousness-driven enterprises can do very well in the marketplace."

— Muhammad Yunus, Banker To The Poor: Micro-Lending and the Battle Against World Poverty

The Spirit of Mutualism

I had a sense that something was missing, though; something was not quite right with the whole picture. CAN was helping a lot of acupuncturists build their own social businesses, but even the relatively progressive combination of social business with a 501(c)(6) nonprofit didn't fully reflect what community acupuncture was about. The more community acupuncture clinics there were, and the busier that they got, the clearer it became that patients weren't just consumers. Beyond paying modest fees for service, patients were constantly making integral contributions. These contributions were usually in the form of time or skills or word of mouth clinic marketing. For tiny, cash-poor, bootstrapped businesses, they were key to community acupuncture's survival. However, the structure of a 501(c)(6) nonprofit business league – what CAN was, technically – didn't include any role for consumers, let alone consumers who were so essential.

I knew this was a huge hole in our structure, because of WCA's own history. In 2002, Skip and I discovered that there was a demand for affordable acupuncture in our neighborhood. But that discovery might never have amounted to anything if I hadn't made another discovery 6 months later– when our 72 year old neighbor Ilse discovered that she wanted to be a receptionist.

Some acupuncturists are talented multi-taskers; I'm not. A few months after the clinic opened, I was giving about 30 treatments a week – 3 times more than any other acupuncturist I knew, and more than anyone suggested was possible outside of a public health setting. I was getting overwhelmed. I had never run an office before, never owned a business before, and didn't know if I was going to be able to support myself and my family with my venture into entrepreneurship. Those uncertainties in the back of my mind sometimes made it hard to figure out the next practical step.

Ilse lived across the street from us and I had been treating her and her husband at home for about a year. Ilse's husband would occasionally express polite skepticism that I would survive in business. He knew I didn't know what I was doing. When I told him I was having a grand opening party, he said, "And when is the grand closing party?" (In his Ukrainian accent, that somehow came across as charming.) One day he joked that I should get Ilse to help me organize my office. Ilse is German and famously organized. We all knew she would order me around and we laughed about it. The longer I tried to run my office by myself, though, the less I minded the thought of being ordered around by someone who had more organizational ability than I did.

Then Ilse's husband died of a heart attack. They had been married 45 years. A week later, I impulsively asked her if she would come and help me get my front office in order. She said yes.

At first, I don't think Ilse had any serious goals beyond getting out of the house. Unlike me, she is a natural extrovert, and sitting at my front desk and greeting my patients was a kind of tonic for her. I was relieved that someone else was answering the phone, because that meant that I didn't have to scurry between patients in the back and a ringing phone in the front. Both of us got our needs met immediately, and it didn't occur to us that there might be more going on than that.

Pretty soon, though, Ilse began making suggestions. She noticed that after acupuncture, people were so relaxed that they often had trouble making their next appointment, as well as writing a check for the appointment they had just had.

They were just as likely to drift out the door without paying. Ilse instituted a policy that patients pay and schedule their next session before a treatment. It worked. A month after Ilse started I made twice as much as I had in any previous month. More people were scheduling because the phone was being answered by a live person (not to mention a warm, friendly, non-harried one) and income was up; I had been forgetting to collect payment from about half of my patients.

Ilse wouldn't let me pay her, though. Initially she thought I was just humoring her, and that I didn't really need help. She changed her mind once she saw the state of my office, but she still maintained that since she had never been a receptionist or worked in a medical office, I shouldn't pay her because she wasn't qualified. I was still giving her acupuncture, so we had a sort of trade. After a few months, she inadvertently admitted that, like many new widows, she had experienced an unexpected drop in income. There was a difference between what her husband's pension paid while he was alive and what it would pay to her after his death. It wouldn't seem like a huge difference, unless you were on a fixed income; in that case it would look exactly like the amount that you spent on groceries.

By this time, it was pretty clear that Ilse's presence in my office was consistently bringing in more business; I was up to 50 visits a week from 30 and no longer losing my mind over the details. We made an arrangement that I would pay her, under the table, a percentage of whatever I brought in. Initially, that percentage added up to grocery money, but eventually, that percentage was not very different from putting her on payroll, which we did. And so I had my first employee. The community acupuncture movement had organically created its first legitimate job. We didn't know that at the time, of course, because there was no community acupuncture movement; there was just Ilse and me, making it up as we went along.

Ilse had invested her time and her skills – skills she didn't realize that she had until she started using them – into a fragile little start-up, and by doing so, she stabilized the fragile start-up into a viable business. 11 years later, the formerly fragile start-up has gross revenues of $740K and employs 27 people. It also provides 40,000 treatments a year to people who otherwise would not be getting acupuncture – a pretty good return on Ilse's investment. By 2007, many new community acupuncture clinics, owned by overwhelmed, disorganized acupuncturists like me, were depending for their survival on the investments of patients like Ilse. Patients were so enthusiastic about the prospect of affordable acupuncture that they were volunteering to help in any way they could: answering phones, doing laundry, hanging up flyers, managing the bookkeeping – for any aspect of the business that didn't involve putting needles in people, some patients were doing for some CAN clinics out of the goodness of their hearts and the desire to see acupuncture remain accessible.

By 2010 we recognized that there was a name for this phenomenon. It's called the *principle of mutual aid*, or the *spirit of mutualism*, and it is the cornerstone of the cooperative movement. Because none of us knew much about business, let alone cooperatives, it didn't dawn on us that what we were doing was more like a cooperative than it was like anything else. We began to investigate whether or not the cooperative movement might be able to help us figure out how to formally recognize the importance of patients' investments.

7 Cooperative Principles
(from the National Cooperative Business Association[9])

Cooperatives around the world generally operate according to the same core principles and values, adopted by the International Co-operative Alliance in 1995. Cooperatives trace the roots of these principles to the first modern cooperative founded in Rochdale, England in 1844.

1. Voluntary and Open Membership
Cooperatives are voluntary organizations, open to all people able to use its services and willing to accept the responsibilities of membership, without gender, social, racial, political or religious discrimination.

2. Democratic Member Control
Cooperatives are democratic organizations controlled by their members – those who buy the goods or use the services of the cooperative – who actively participate in setting policies and making decisions.

3. Members' Economic Participation
Members contribute equally to, and democratically control, the capital of the cooperative. This benefits members in proportion to the business they conduct with the cooperative rather than on the capital invested.

4. Autonomy and Independence
Cooperatives are autonomous, self-help organizations controlled by their members. If the co-op enters into agreements with other organizations or raises capital from external sources, it is done so based on terms that ensure democratic control by the members and maintains the cooperative's autonomy.

---

[9] http://usa2012.coop/about-co-ops/7-cooperative-principles

5. Education, Training and Information
Cooperatives provide education and training for members, elected representatives, managers and employees so they can contribute effectively to the development of their cooperative. Members also inform the general public about the nature and benefits of cooperatives.

6. Cooperation among Cooperatives
Cooperatives serve their members most effectively and strengthen the cooperative movement by working together through local, national, regional and international structures.

7. Concern for Community
While focusing on member needs, cooperatives work for the sustainable development of communities through policies and programs accepted by the members.

Multi-Stakeholder Cooperative

Cooperatives are complex business entities. It didn't seem feasible to try to get all of the clinics represented by CAN to convert from LLCs or partnerships or sole proprietorships into cooperatives. For one thing, it would cost too much for all the clinics to hire the specialized lawyers and accountants they would need. Furthermore, it wasn't immediately obvious what kind of cooperative business model we would choose. Were we consumer cooperatives (like food co-ops) or worker cooperatives (like bakeries and printing presses) or producer cooperatives (like dairy farmers)? What made it hard to figure out was the sheer simplicity of the community acupuncture model. We needed almost nothing in terms of materials – needles, cotton balls, a room full of second-hand recliners – and we made just enough money to pay ourselves. We charged our patients just enough to keep the whole thing running. All that "restful nothingness" and "the body healing itself," not to mention the social business aspect of just breaking even, didn't translate very well into the cooperative language of patronage and dividends. In some ways, what we were doing barely involved money at all. And yet, in order to do it, we needed to make a living; and yet, the core of our economic relationship with our patients was obviously cooperative. What to do?

Fortunately, cooperatives are enormously flexible. We learned that people form them for all kinds of purposes. They are especially useful in economic situations that have some element of market failure. (Learning this was the fact that made me the most hopeful.) For instance, many rural parts of the U.S would have had no electricity or telephone service if residents had not formed cooperatives. It was simply not profitable enough for big power companies or telephone companies to serve relatively far-flung places with relatively few people. It wasn't worth it to the big companies to provide electricity, but it was absolutely worth it to those relatively few people in those relatively far-flung places to HAVE electricity; it was worth the trouble for them to organize themselves into a cooperative in order to get what they needed. The market may have failed them, but they didn't fail each other. That was exactly the commitment that the patients and the acupuncturists of the CAN were expressing, daily, in their clinics.

As we researched cooperatives, we came across a relatively new type that seemed to reflect all the important elements we were trying to encompass: a multi-stakeholder cooperative. Instead of being solely a consumer cooperative (created to provide goods or services at affordable rates to people who otherwise couldn't access them), or solely a worker's cooperative (created to provide stable jobs in a market not otherwise inclined to provide them), a multi-stakeholder cooperative includes both consumers and workers. It might seem that consumers and workers would have economic interests that are too far apart to allow them to cooperate, but in reality, a situation in which a market is truly failing means that consumers and workers have a lot in common. If a service is not available at a price that sufficient numbers of people can afford, not enough revenue will be generated to create stable jobs providing that service. If there are no stable jobs providing that service, how can consumers have reliable access to it? Neither consumers nor workers are getting what they need, and so they have nothing to lose and everything to gain by uniting voluntarily in order to create economic structures that can meet their respective needs. Many cooperatives invoke the phrase, "better together" and this is just as true of multi-stakeholder enterprises.

Often, people join cooperatives because by doing so they get a better price on goods or services. Some cooperatives are buying clubs in which people pool their money to access wholesale prices. A multi-stakeholder co-op is a little different, because it is not only focused on short-term economic benefits (though it usually includes a few); rather, it is designed to build a long-term, stable economic relationship based on fair treatment for everybody. We found a helpful manual, *Solidarity as a Business Model*.[10] In it, Margaret Lund, of the Cooperative Development Center at Kent State University, describes multi-stakeholder co-ops as "transformational rather than transactional." If ever a field needs to prioritize big picture economic transformation over narrowly self-interested transactions, it is acupuncture in America. The community acupuncture business model already provided a pretty good deal on acupuncture to a hundred thousand or so patients; multi-stakeholder cooperative for acupuncture would not provide those people with a better deal. The purpose would be to anchor the community acupuncture movement in a more stable economic foundation than that of a few hundred bootstrapping acupuncturist entrepreneurs, loosely connected to each other through a professional association.

By the time we discovered the concept of a multi-stakeholder cooperative, the community acupuncture business model had proved over and over, that in big cities and in small towns, it could deliver affordable acupuncture to large numbers of people and create living wage jobs for acupuncturists. The problem was that the business model was expressed in separate small businesses that were, unfortunately, small and separate. They were each relatively fragile because most depended on a single owner. If something happened to that individual, the clinic would disappear. Although these

10   http://www.community-wealth.org/content/solidarity-business-model-multi-stakeholder-cooperatives-manual

businesses had many common needs, they had no way of joining together economically either to reinforce each other, or to access the economies of scale that benefit and stabilize bigger businesses. And while many patients benefited greatly from community acupuncture clinics, because most of them were individually owned by acupuncturists and were not profitable in a conventional sense, no economic mechanism existed for patients to invest in them as businesses to help them stabilize and grow.

There were thousands of community acupuncture patients who might not have money to invest in growing community acupuncture clinics, but they had other resources that were infinitely valuable – skills, time and enthusiasm – and they were investing them, every day. We knew that the community acupuncture movement was not going to appeal to a typical venture capitalist as an investment opportunity; community acupuncture doesn't look like a good investment from a narrow financial perspective any more than providing electricity to rural areas in the 1930s looked like a good investment to the big power companies. The natural investors in the community acupuncture movement were the patients and the acupuncturists; the return on their investment was, respectively, affordable acupuncture and dependable jobs.

As we reflected on what the movement needed, we realized it wasn't about making individual clinics into cooperatives, it was about officially recognizing the cooperative relationship between acupuncturists and patients, and creating infrastructure for ourselves. Profits usually pay for infrastructure, but we didn't have any profits. We had already proved our ability to build things with very modest resources. We began to think of a cooperative as a way to build a super-structure around the movement and to organize the resources that we had more efficiently. The primary resource that we had was goodwill. Every clinic was like a spring coming out of the ground, out of a community, bubbling up with goodwill. But because the springs were small and separate, some of the goodwill just drained away. Couldn't we build a reservoir to capture the goodwill that the whole movement generated?

A small group of community acupuncturists spent a year drawing up the blueprints for our reservoir. On March 18, 2011, the **People's Organization of Community Acupuncture**, a new multi-stakeholder cooperative, formally incorporated in the state of Oregon.

POCA (get it?)

POCA is an international multi-stakeholder cooperative with four membership categories. Each category represents a type of stakeholder: someone or something that benefits if the movement grows and succeeds. The categories are: patients/community members (individual humans), acupuncturists/acupuncture students (also individual humans), community acupuncture clinics (business entities), and organizations (such as Cleanwell[11], a company that makes natural hand sanitizer (POCA clinics go through tanker trucks of Cleanwell). The cooperative creates a structure for those entities to relate to each other in a spirit of mutual aid and self-help. POCA is not a vehicle for financial investment; there is no patronage, no dividends, and no expectation that membership will lead to any individual financial benefits at all. Membership in POCA is about creating a new – cooperative – economic foundation for acupuncture.

POCA is able to do many of the things that CAN did successfully: host a website where community acupuncturists can have conversations and share information, put on annual conferences, and generally cultivate a spirit of camaraderie and support in the erstwhile isolated, lonely acupuncture profession. As a cooperative, though, POCA demanded a higher level of organization; where CAN was loose and informal (we changed our bylaws whenever we felt like it, and never had a real election), POCA was bureaucratic – in a good way.

For years, people had been asking CAN about micro-lending, but there were a lot of difficulties with a 501(c)(6) nonprofit loaning money. By virtue of being a cooperative, POCA was instantly able to function as a micro-lending institution, since

[11] http://www.cleanwelltoday.com/

members of a cooperative can loan money to other members. In December 2012, POCA issued its first microloan to start a new community acupuncture clinic in Guelph, Ontario.

Because POCA is a cooperative, it has to have elections, which means that it needs more of a structure for participation than CAN had. This one requirement released a flood of creative thinking about governance (which, previously, we had mostly avoided thinking about), and led to a novel way of organizing POCA's administrative volunteers, based on a system called sociocracy. POCA's governance structure consists of several semi-autonomous, self-organizing, interlocking "circles" (similar to committees).

One of them, Clinic Success, is a circle whose mission is to "provide support to any POCA member through all phases of clinic development from start up to sustainability, and address the clinic success needs of members by using the wealth of experience and best practices of POCA member clinics." In other words, POCA has a free peer mentor program for members who own or work in community acupuncture clinics. For years CAN discussed standardizing and centralizing "Community Acupuncture 101" workshops, but didn't make much progress; POCA's Events Circle got this process underway immediately. There are also circles devoted to publications and the website. POCA produces materials to help clinics implement the model: operations manuals, step-by-step guides to opening clinics, templates for forms and for physical layout, and wikis. New acupuncturist members often express relief at not having to reinvent the wheel.

Perhaps most importantly, though, POCA officially established and recognized the participation of patients. According to the bylaws, patients are represented on the Board of Directors as elected members. Just as members in a cooperative can loan money to each other, members in a cooperative can contribute non-financial resources such as time and skills to each other, for the purpose of strengthening the cooperative as a whole. Patient and community members in POCA, once they sign a few forms, are able to volunteer either for their local clinic or for the administrative circles of POCA itself – and hundreds of them do. Thus people are able to become investors, even when they do not have money to invest. Their time and energy are tangible, valuable resources; the return on their investment is affordable acupuncture.

This structural change was a huge improvement. When the only structure we had was CAN's 501(c)(6) nonprofit, the emphasis on having a professional organization for acupuncturists made it seem as if 1) the professional acupuncturists were the only ones doing the work, or the only ones whose work was important; and 2) the professional acupuncturists just happened to be providing affordable acupuncture out of lofty humanitarian idealism rather than a pragmatic desire to earn a living. Having a cooperative as the primary institution reflects the reality that, when it comes to affordable acupuncture, patients and acupuncturists depend on each other absolutely. Community acupuncture is not charity; it's self-help within our communities. A multi-stakeholder cooperative provides the means by which the natural investors can participate in the community acupuncture movement, as well as for individual clinics to join together in a more coherent economic whole.

Cooperatives are flexible things, but experts on cooperatives have commented that POCA pushes the boundaries. One of them described our structure as "out on the ragged edge of organizational development." We like to think of POCA as innovative (as opposed to just wacky). But the most important thing about POCA is that it works for us. It does what the community acupuncture movement needs it to do. Our accountant, who specializes in cooperatives, described POCA as "a bank for social and financial capital." There is no generally agreed upon definition of social capital. We think of it as the power of relationships; the willingness of people to give their time, energy, and attention to the needs of the community acupuncture movement; and the goodwill that makes collective progress possible. Because most of the people who are involved in the cooperative don't have much money, we have a lot more social capital than we have financial capital. The best thing about social capital, though, is that the more of it you use, the more of it you have.[12]

POCA works as a cooperative, even though its structure is unusual, because it is essentially a vehicle for people who do not have much money to empower each other. When you think about it, it is exactly what community acupuncture is, too. Acupuncture itself needs so little to work: needles, cotton balls, and stillness. Community acupuncture is about making this core of restful, healing nothingness available to more and more people who need it. If the nature of our technical work in the cooperative were different – if we were trying to run a steel mill – we would need more financial capital, and there would be more questions about profits. As an industry in the West, however, acupuncture has proved itself over the last few decades to be, for most acupuncturists, unprofitable. In a sense, what POCA is doing is accepting that there is no financial profit to be extracted from the practice of acupuncture: there is only social good, in the form of affordable treatments and stable jobs. And if there is only social good, why not put our energy into trying to share it?

---

[12] http://www.yesmagazine.org/issues/reclaiming-the-commons/the-cornucopia-of-the-commons

POCA's Mission and Vision

Our mission is to work cooperatively to increase accessibility to and availability of affordable group acupuncture treatments.

POCA, as a multi-stakeholder co-op, is designed to build a long-term, stable economic relationship based on fair treatment for everybody. Multi-stakeholder cooperatives recognize that producers and consumers are mutually dependent on one another, and that the health of the relationship between these groups is connected to the health of the larger community and economy.

Our vision is to:

- make community acupuncture as widely available as possible.
- establish affordable acupuncture training and continuing education programs.
- establish best practices for the operation of sustainable community acupuncture clinics.
- create job stability for community acupuncture employees, staff, and clinic owners.
- build healthy relationships and foster collaboration among our practitioners, staff, patients, and communities.
- establish micro-lending programs, scholarship funds, insurance/benefits programs, and further financial support to POCA members.
- ease entry into the practice of acupuncture and work with legislators to ensure safety and reasonable regulation.
- develop research that is useful to POCA clinics, patients, and practitioners.
- build alliances with organizations that build community and foster sustainable economies.
- sustain POCA as a robust, flourishing cooperative.

POCA Tech

Another significant difference between CAN and POCA is that CAN was primarily ideological, and POCA is primarily economic. CAN was about rallying acupuncturists to consider social justice in their practices; POCA is about organizing acupuncturists, patients, and community supporters to create a sustainable, cooperative foundation for affordable acupuncture.

CAN had a lot of fun being ideological. After I was fired from *Acupuncture Today* for having dangerous ideas, the public platform for community acupuncture moved to CAN's website, especially to its blog, which we gleefully titled "Prick, Prod and Provoke." (If you look up "to needle" in a thesaurus, you will find that definitions include "to tease or annoy," synonyms include "aggravate, badger, bedevil, bother, examine, goad, irk, irritate, nettle, pester, plague, prick, prod, and provoke.") By then we were accustomed to hearing regular laments from other acupuncturists that we were "devaluing an ancient and honorable profession," "debasing the traditions," and (most memorably) "lowering Acupuncture and Chinese Medicine respectability in the minds of the media, health care community, patients, practitioners and future generations in America forever." We were accused not only of being communists, but terrorists. We figured that if we were publicly writing about what we were doing, we were surely aggravating somebody; so we might as well enjoy it.

From the late 1990s onward, one of the major issues occupying the rest of the profession in the US was the question of what degree one should have. Acupuncturists had begun with no degrees, progressed to diplomas and certificates, and then to Master's degrees. Some practitioners felt strongly that

Master's degrees weren't professional enough and that the entry-level degree should be a doctorate. Then acupuncturists could be called "Doctor." There was a public debate, and CAN joined the fray.

We argued that many acupuncturists already couldn't repay their student loans, and the degrees we had were already bloated. We argued that patients didn't care about titles; they cared about safe, effective, affordable acupuncture. We accused the rest of the profession of being shameless status-seekers. They responded that yes, the degrees *were* inflated, and that's why they needed to be upgraded to a doctorate; you couldn't continue to cap such a distended curriculum with a mere "Master's." They claimed that a doctorate wouldn't cost more than a Master's degree, due to the bloat. (Nobody besides us suggested addressing the bloat itself.) They claimed that hospitals would hire unemployed acupuncturists en masse if only those acupuncturists had the right degrees. They accused us of being "LOUD MOUTHED UNDEREDUCATED OVER OPINIONATED MISINFORMED LOW LEVEL PRACTITIONERS." (All caps theirs.) We wrote rude haikus[13] about them.

degree lined bird cage
bright colors loud and organized
squawking "pretty-bird"

As entertaining as this was, it wasn't getting us anywhere. Moral indignation, off-color poetry, and Internet snark are not solutions to an economic problem. In the course of various arguments online, the most important thing that we learned was that the cost of tuition and the accessibility of acupuncture education was all about the market, and the

---

[13] https://www.pocacoop.com/prick-prod-provoke/post/the-zang-fools-15th-annual-fpd-haiku-competition

market, as far as the bureaucracy of the profession was concerned, was in the hands of the acupuncture schools. Nobody was going to step in and intervene. If schools wanted to offer streamlined, affordable, accessible degrees, then those degrees would exist; if they didn't, they wouldn't. We realized that the solution was for POCA to open a school.

In December 2011, we formed an educational nonprofit and christened it the POCA Technical Institute.[14] We drafted a business plan that kept tuition low by relying heavily on working POCA acupuncturists volunteering as teachers and mentors for POCA Tech students.

POCA Tech is the educational arm of POCA. Since POCA's goal is to make acupuncture available and accessible to as many people as possible, and to support those providing acupuncture to create stable and sustainable businesses and jobs, POCA Tech's aim is to provide the cooperative with educational programs that back up its mission. Its first goal is to create entry-level training programs for acupuncturists that are affordable to prospective students of ordinary incomes.

We realized fairly quickly, though, that it wasn't enough just to create an affordable acupuncture training program. If we really wanted to create a new economic foundation for acupuncture, the most important aspect of POCA Tech shouldn't be to offer an affordable education for acupuncturists, or even to teach community acupuncture. We didn't want an acupuncture school just to have an acupuncture school, even if it was a cheap one. The acupuncture profession is in deep trouble largely because the process of educating acupuncturists has eclipsed the business of doing acupuncture. If we are going to educate acupuncturists, we have to be sure to do it in context.

---

[14] http://www.pocatech.org

The most important thing about POCA Tech should be its role within the collective structure of POCA as a cooperative that includes patients, genuinely supportive acupuncturists, and future employers and mentors for graduates. POCA Tech should be a means to an end, not an end in itself. The only people we want in POCA Tech are people who are willing to be as collectively minded as the rest of POCA, who think of themselves as co-op members before they think of themselves as students. Almost everybody in the acupuncture profession – as well as thousands or millions of potential patients who need acupuncture but can't get it – are suffering because of the lack of infrastructure for acupuncturists. Everybody wants the benefits of more infrastructure, but most acupuncturists don't want to think about acupuncture as anything other than an exclusively personal, individual experience. In order to help as many patients as possible, POCA is devoted to building real infrastructure for community acupuncturists. We can't squander our hard-won social capital on educating people who don't care about the collective, or who only care about it as far as it benefits themselves. The purpose of POCA Tech must be to grow the next generation of acupuncturists who will pitch in with the hard work of building a new foundation for acupuncture, which means growing the cooperative.

So POCA Tech's new Board of Directors passed a resolution:

The purpose of POCA Tech is to educate and train members of the POCA cooperative to work as licensed acupuncturists in POCA clinics.

The market rate for acupuncture education leading to licensure ranges from $10,000 to $25,000 per year for tuition. Our goal is to keep POCA Tech's tuition under $6,000 per year. This drastic reduction in cost is possible only because of the generous contributions of time, energy and funds to POCA Tech from members of the POCA Cooperative. Members have made these contributions with the faith that they will be used only for the purpose of providing well-trained workers to current and future clinics of the Cooperative.

In order to ensure that the contributions of the members of the Cooperative are used appropriately, the Board requires that the following conditions be met:

1) Admissions: application process

Admission to POCA Tech shall be limited to applicants who have been members of the POCA Cooperative for at least 3 months. Applicants shall provide evidence that they have used those 3 months to familiarize themselves with the structure and function of the POCA Cooperative, especially its online forums.

Applicants to POCA Tech are strongly encouraged to provide at least one letter of recommendation from a current POCA member.

Applicants to POCA Tech shall provide evidence that they clearly understand the responsibilities, obligations, and expected compensation of the position for which they are training: licensed acupuncturist in a POCA clinic.

Preference in admissions shall be given to applicants who have provided volunteer service to the POCA Cooperative, either as a working member in a POCA clinic or as an administrative volunteer to one of the Cooperative Circles.

2) Enrollment

Once accepted to POCA Tech, a condition of enrollment shall be that students sign an agreement that they will upon graduation:
1) obtain a license to practice acupuncture; and
2) work for at least three years after obtaining their license either as an
acupuncturist employee of an existing POCA clinic, or work to open a new POCA clinic as an acupuncturist owner.

3) Clinical Mentorship

Students shall be required, as part of their clinical training, to find an experienced POCA acupuncturist member to consult with. If possible, this mentor shall live in the region where the student ultimately plans to practice.

4) Graduation

A condition of graduation from POCA Tech shall be that students produce a business plan either for an existing POCA clinic that describes how they will be employed, or for a new POCA clinic which they will open. Each student's business plan shall be reviewed by a committee of POCA members drawn from the region in which they plan to work. Students shall graduate only when the committee has approved their business plan.

We hope to open POCA Tech in early 2014. Creating a school is certainly much more demanding than writing rude haikus, but it's ultimately more fulfilling.

Co-ops, Fractals, and You

There's always a tension between the individual and the collective. That tension can be like a dance, a creative balance, or a constantly recalibrating vibration – or it can be brittle and fraught, like a string stretched to the breaking point and constantly on the edge of unraveling. All cooperatives have to learn how to manage this tension in a healthy, dynamic way. POCA is no exception.

Patients don't have to join POCA to get acupuncture in a POCA clinic. Acupuncturists don't have to join POCA to use the community acupuncture model. The idea of community acupuncture is out in the world, and people can do whatever they want to do with it. (Of course, some people are inevitably stretching the model to the breaking point, doing things that make me wince.) If you want, you can take a completely individual approach to community acupuncture, and look at it only in terms of how it is useful to you. I'm going to argue, though, that to approach community acupuncture this way is to miss out on the best, and most essential, part of it.

What is the purpose of acupuncture today, in the West? If you read acupuncture textbooks, it's clear that acupuncture was intended to treat a vast range of ailments. At the time these treatments were developed, acupuncture was the best intervention on hand. Today, however, there are more effective ways to treat schizophrenia and dysentery –to name two examples; and of course, the widespread availability of clean water, toilets, antibiotics and emergency rooms has changed everything, mostly for the better. Why do we need acupuncture now?

We overuse high-tech medicine in this culture. We overuse antibiotics, with disastrous consequences. Our desire for quick fixes has left us at the mercy of the pharmaceutical industry, which seems to have no mercy. The widespread availability of a low-tech, inexpensive therapy for pain and stress that is virtually free of side effects is a blessing. But I think acupuncture has even more to give the West than that: it offers us healing from our rigid, dualistic perspective.

We don't suffer only from our individual ailments; we suffer from our collective ones, too. We are inclined, in the West, to chop things up into little pieces in our heads and then to try to triumph over them. We love dualities and we believe in them unquestioningly a lot of the time: good/bad, health/illness, mind/body, strong/weak, victory/defeat, fixed/broken. We don't leave any room for mystery. But life itself doesn't work that way. It doesn't fit into neat dualities, and it's full of mysteries and paradoxes. Chopping things up in our heads and believing that the resulting pieces are real, and that we can know everything there is to know about them, alienates us from the processes of life, especially its healing processes. We take an aggressive, dominating, mechanistic approach to our bodies all the time, and so we become alienated from them. Acupuncture relieves that kind of alienation.

One of the things that you learn pretty quickly when you are working in a community acupuncture clinic, whether you are an acupuncturist in the treatment room, a receptionist at the front desk, or a regular POCA volunteer, is that you can't hold on to the usual dualisms when you are faced with day-to-day life in the clinic. Health and illness are not separate, distinct states; you can see that in the people who come in for treatment. Most people are on a continuum somewhere between health and illness, not firmly on one side or the other, trying to make the best of it. Acupuncture is not powerful enough to force somebody over the line from illness to health in one fell swoop, like surgery. There's a lot of hanging out in the in-between in a community acupuncture clinic. There, you can see also that the mind and the body are not separate. People's mental states have enormous influence on their physical states, and vice versa. Spending time in a community acupuncture clinic, whether as a volunteer or a patient or a staff member, helps wear down the edges of all those hard mental dualisms. You experience life in a softer way.

I think that softening, that breaking down of dualism, is a large part of why so many people feel that our clinic spaces are healing to them. What St. Paul said about love is true about acupuncture: it's patient, it's kind, it doesn't insist on its own way, it's not boastful. It's gentle and slow and it tries to help things work out instead of forcing them. It depends on an acceptance of mystery. When people get acupuncture, aspects of themselves that were cut apart by our culture are able to grow back together in the stillness and peace of the treatment room. The mind and the body, the conscious and the unconscious, get closer together.

The core idea of yin and yang theory is that opposites are complementary; the original images for yin and yang were the shady side of the hill and the sunny side of the hill, respectively – but there is only one hill. Nobody cut the hill in half; the sun is just moving over it. When people can afford to get regular acupuncture, they get to experience the different aspects of themselves more like a hill with the sun moving over it, and less like a lot of chopped-up pieces with labels and diagnoses. Acupuncture restores a sense of internal relationship, and allows people to feel more connected to themselves.

In Western medicine, there's often a sense that the goal is to triumph over illness: to diagnose it, to beat it and to win. But so often in community acupuncture, we are treating people who are not going to triumph over their conditions; they have to manage them. Whether it's a chronic condition, or age, or stress, or some difficult aspect of life, there isn't going to be any clear-cut triumphant moment where you get to declare victory – whatever that is. Because acupuncture is gentle and gradual, people who are getting it regularly are embracing the need to care for themselves as opposed to beating their illnesses – even if they wouldn't quite use those words, that's still what they're doing.

In fact, as an acupuncturist, even if you do "beat" one condition, often another one pops up, or your patient's left knee still hurts for no reason you can figure out, or just when his shoulder pain was finally going away, he gets into another bike accident and breaks his arm. A lot of what community acupuncture clinics do is to help people accept and work with whatever it is: stress, pain, disability, limitations, illness, terminal illness, loss. We encourage and support and accompany people in working with whatever it is that their lives have given them to work with. We try to get out of the way and let them connect with their own inner resources, their own source of healing – which doesn't mean that everything gets fixed. Probably the main thing community acupuncture is doing is trying to give ordinary people a better quality of life. That's not a dualistic undertaking. It's not a win-lose kind of scenario. It's creative and it's hopeful and it emphasizes working with what you've got. Of course, it helps immensely that acupuncture itself almost always gives people more energy, better sleep, a lift in their mood, a reduction in their stress: the humblest things are sometimes the most important.

We don't believe that acupuncture is a magical cure for every problem. We do believe that people should be able to try it to find out for themselves if it will help them. Along with trying to give ordinary people a better quality of life, the community acupuncture movement is trying to equalize people's access to acupuncture as an option to manage their health. Being lower-class generally means that you automatically have fewer positive options; your choices shrink. Chronic health problems, especially chronic pain, can mean that your whole life shrinks: you are able to do fewer things, engage with fewer people, and have fewer possibilities. Under these conditions, giving people the option of trying something positive, giving them back a choice, is itself empowering. And we also believe that equalizing access is beneficial not only to lower-class people and people facing chronic health problems, but to everyone. A society where access to positive choices is more equal is one that values fairness: a healthier society.

A cooperative, especially a multi-stakeholder cooperative that doesn't make enough money to issue dividends, is very similar. It breaks down the dualism of consumers and producers, customers and business owners. It makes something without having to make profits. It makes something out of what conventional business wisdom considers nothing – out of many small contributions of time, energy and goodwill. It gives people who don't often have choices the choice to participate in something positive. When patients can get affordable acupuncture, and acupuncturists can make a living wage, everybody's quality of life gets better. POCA's goals are modest in the same way that community acupuncture's goals are modest. We're not trying to triumph over Western medicine and show the world all the ways that it's wrong. We're not demanding that acupuncturists be given the same status as doctors. We're not trying to win at the business of health care, or be something important; we just want to give everyone a better quality of life, to open up access to positive choices. Just as acupuncture empowers people to help themselves with respect to their health, a cooperative empowers people to help themselves around the economics of health care.

This is why the community acupuncture movement is a fractal: the same elements of the pattern repeat at each level. Acupuncture is a creative, nurturing, simple, empowering, non-dualistic way to help your body. It uses your own internal resources rather than looking outward for something to fix you. The community acupuncture business model is a creative, nurturing, simple, empowering, non-dualistic way to provide acupuncture in communities that can't afford conventional rates. It's not really for-profit, but it's not a nonprofit either; it uses resources that are immediately available, like cheap space and used recliners. You don't have to look outward for an insurance company, or the government, to pay for acupuncture treatments for people of ordinary incomes. We really don't know how acupuncture works, but we know it does. The POCA Cooperative is a creative, nurturing, simple, empowering, non-dualistic way to make health care work better. We're not waiting for the government or the health care industry to fix the economics of acupuncture for us. It doesn't matter so much whether we are consumers or providers, because we're trying to do something transformational together. Just as we don't know how acupuncture works, it is something of a mystery how POCA achieves all that it does, given our financial circumstances. Even though we don't have much money, POCA uses what we already have, which is each other. At every level, the fractal gives us dignity and hope.

You can participate in the fractal at any level you choose. When you join POCA as a member you participate in the fractal at a level where you can see it doing its beautiful organic fractal-thing. Besides enjoying the taste of a broccoli floret, you get to see the stalk – and you get to help it grow.

Some people who study fractals argue that their existence proves that there is a force in the universe that counteracts entropy. The final word might not be that everything breaks down into little pieces and ultimately falls apart, despite what we believe. The existence of fractals – rivers, ferns, broccoli, and POCA – suggests that life loves connectivity and self-organizing structures.

Unequal access to resources, an aggressive and mechanistic approach to the body, greed and fear – all these elements in health care separate people from each other, and separate people from themselves. We can choose to be part of something that is moving in a different direction, though: towards more equal access, towards cooperation, towards trust in our own inner resources, towards deeper connection with ourselves and each other. What better way to respond to the broken state of health care than to become part of a fractal, part of the community acupuncture movement?

Join **POCA**.

Sources

Needles, Herbs, Gods and Ghosts: China, Healing and the West to 1848, Linda L. Barnes, © 2005 by the President and Fellows of Harvard College

The Little Red Book of Working Class Acupuncture, 10ᵗʰ Anniversary Edition, Lisa Rohleder and Skip Van Meter, © 2012, Working Class Acupuncture, Portland, OR

The Web That Has No Weaver: Understanding Chinese Medicine, Ted Kaptchuk OMD, © 1983, Congdon & Weed, Inc., Chicago, Illinois

Creating a World without Poverty: Social Business and the Future of Capitalism, Muhammad Yunus, © 2007, Public Affairs, New York, New York

The People's Organization of Community Acupuncture, http://www.pocacoop.com